ELAINE LaLANNE SHOWS YOU HOW TO BREAK YOUR BAD HABITS . . . AND GIVE YOURSELF THE GIFT OF GOOD HEALTH

If you like to have:	*Try this instead:*
*Toast, butter, jelly	*2 No, No-No Muffins (no salt, sugar, or oil, just great taste and only 175 calories)
*Flapjacks and sausage	*Norwegian Waffles (sinfully good) & Quickie Applesauce (homemade & yummy)
*Hamburger and french fries	*Marinated Chicken Sandwich on Sourdough Roll with Salad of Green & Gold (a gourmet treat)
*Steak and potatoes	*Steak & Veggies (surprise! you don't have to go meatless)
*Chocolate cake	*Pleasing Peach Meringues (a five-star dessert)

Eating Right For a New You

Peak Nutrition for Fitness After Fifty

ELAINE LaLANNE is the author of three previous books on fitness, *Fitness After Fifty Workout, Dynastride! A Complete Walking Program for Fitness After Fifty*, and *Fitness After Fifty*. She has been an advocate for health and fitness with her husband Jack LaLanne for more than 35 years. The LaLannes live in San Luis Obispo, California.

Eating Right

For A New You

Peak Nutrition for Fitness After Fifty

Elaine LaLanne

with Richard Benyo

Foreword by Jack LaLanne

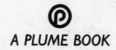

A PLUME BOOK

PLUME
Published by the Penguin Group
Penguin Books USA Inc., 375 Hudson Street,
New York, New York 10014, U.S.A.
Penguin Books Ltd, 27 Wrights Lane,
London W8 5TZ, England
Penguin Books Australia Ltd, Ringwood,
Victoria, Australia
Penguin Books Canada Ltd, 10 Alcorn Avenue,
Toronto, Ontario, Canada M4V 3B2
Penguin Books (N.Z.) Ltd, 182–190 Wairau Road,
Auckland 10, New Zealand

Penguin Books Ltd, Registered Offices:
Harmondsworth, Middlesex, England

First published by Plume, an imprint of New American Library, a division of Penguin Books
USA Inc.

First Printing, October, 1992
10 9 8 7 6 5 4 3 2

 REGISTERED TRADEMARK—MARCA REGISTRADA

Library of Congress Cataloging-in-Publication Data:
LaLanne, Elaine, 1926–
    Eating right for a new you : peak nutrition for fitness after fifty / Elaine LaLanne with
Richard Benyo : foreword by Jack LaLanne.
        p.   cm.
    Includes index.
    ISBN 0-452-26910-5
    1. Middle aged persons—Nutrition.   I. Benyo, Richard.
II. Title.
RA784.L33   1992
613.2′084′4—dc20   92-53552
                                                              CIP

PRINTED IN THE UNITED STATES OF AMERICA
Set in Clearface
Designed by Leonard Telesca

A NOTE TO THE READER
The ideas, procedures, and suggestions contained in this book are not intended as a
substitute for consulting with your physician. All matters regarding your health require
medical supervision.

In memory of my mother,
Betty Sylvia Michaelson Rorem

Acknowledgments

Dr. Gale Shemwell-Rudolph, a Ph.D. in nutrition from UCLA, and a consultant in nutrition and food science, for her invaluable input while reviewing our manuscript;

Carolyn Katzin, M.S. in nutrition at the School of Public Health at UCLA, for her time and patience in making numerous calibrations and calculations to assure that our breakdowns of calories, proteins, carbohydrates, and fats are accurate;

Terry Ganes, a good friend and neighbor who was an invaluable partner in the kitchen while we cooked and sampled this book's recipes;

Brenda Rodriques, my secretary, whose assistance not only from the creative side but in typing, retyping, and keeping a constantly evolving manuscript on track, was invaluable;

Jack LaLanne, who taught me years ago that there's more to a good meal than meat and potatoes, and who continues to inspire me; and

Richard Benyo, my long-running collaborator, for tolerating all my shortcuts.

And special thanks to all those who were kind enough to share their very special recipes with my very special readers.

Contents

Foreword
by Jack LaLanne

It seems that everywhere I go, people say to me: "You must have had good genes. Your mother and father must have been very healthy people."

Nothing could be further from the truth.

It seemed that early in my life my mother and father were constantly sick. I also remember that my uncle and grandfather were constantly ailing.

As a child I was a sugarholic and was sick all the time. By the age of fifteen, I was a junk food junkie. I had boils and pimples and needed arch supports and glasses. I frequently had blinding headaches so bad I used to pound my head against the wall because I couldn't stand the pain. I was getting failing grades in school. I was thinking about suicide.

At the age of fifteen I was so sick I had to drop out of school for six months.

It was during this time that a neighbor, Mrs. Joy, suggested that my mother take me to a health lecture in Oakland, California. I didn't want to go, but my mother dragged me along.

That lecture became a turning point in my life. This man, Paul Bragg, was inspiring. He said that I could be reborn, meaning that if I would obey Nature's laws, improve my eating habits, and take up an exercise program, I could change my body.

I immediately stopped eating white flour and white sugar products, ate foods in their natural state as often as possible, and joined the local YMCA. I was inspired! My goal was to have a healthy body, play sports, and be a good student.

I bought a copy of *Gray's Anatomy* and read it cover to cover. I went back to school, became captain of the football team, an A.A.U. wrestling champion in my weight class for the state of California, sold dates and nuts on the side as a part-time job, and preached nutrition to my classmates. I also set up a gym in my backyard. I built exercise equipment of my own invention. Firemen and police officers came to my backyard to work out on my equipment. This was while I was still a high school student. I would put them on individual programs aimed at their specific exercise needs and I'd also put them on healthy meal menus, while continually checking their progress.

In college I wanted to become a medical doctor, but after thinking about it gave up that idea because I felt it was more important to help people before they became sick. I opened the very first physical culture studio in the country. In 1936 there was no place a person could go to work out with weights other than boxing and wrestling gyms, which were called sweat boxes. I wanted people to have a nice atmosphere in which they could work out, a place with rugs on the floors, plants all around, clean block-glass showers, steam baths, and health foods. So I opened just such a place on Fourteenth Street in Oakland, paying $45 a month rent.

The gym was on the second floor and the health food store was on the first floor. People made fun of me. They called me a muscleman, crackpot, health nut. Doctors told people that they shouldn't go to that Jack LaLanne's or they'd get musclebound.

I went to the local high schools in a tight T-shirt and talked to the skinny kids about building their muscles, and to the heavy kids about eating right and working out. I had to sell the parents on the idea. When the kids started getting good results, the parents began coming, too. I even earned a degree in chiropractic in my attempts to further understand the workings of the human body.

From time to time, to keep clients interested in working out, I would invent a new piece of equipment. That is how the first weight selector, leg-extension machine, and the first pulley-based exercise machine came into being. In those days I never thought to patent anything and now those concepts are used all over the world.

On the nutrition side, many of my students didn't want to take the time to eat breakfast, so in the late 1950s I worked with a biochemist and developed one of the first powdered protein drinks, called Instant Breakfast.

Everyone seems to have an idea about nutrition. Someone will say, "Eat this!" Another will say, "Don't eat this!" or "Don't eat that!" Or they'll say, "Combine this with that" or "Don't ever combine this with that" or "Eat two meals a day" or "Eat three meals a day" or "Eat six meals a day" or "Eat more carbohydrates" or "Eat more protein." I've been studying nutrition for more than sixty years now and I can see why there is so much confusion. I have tried about every diet there is. When I was training for the Mr. America contest years ago, the big thing was to bulk up by eating a lot of red meat. I was eating two to three pounds of red meat a day. I wasn't feeling that great while on this regime and discovered it was because I was getting *too much* protein from animal sources. For a while I went so far as to experiment with drinking steer blood that I got from the local slaughterhouse. I should explain why I did this.

Being interested in athletics, I read about different people all over the world and researched the sources of their athletic abilities. I was fascinated with the Masai tribe in Kenya, Africa. For the most part, they were herders engaged in cattle raising, but they were also noted for their great athletic accomplishments and their great height. They lived on milk, blood, and meat they took from their cattle. The adults would drink straight blood and the children half blood and half goat's milk, and they were one of the healthiest and longest-lived tribes in Africa.

So I got the bright idea that what was good for them ought to be good for me. Why not try it? So every morning I went down to the slaughterhouse and drank a quart of steer blood. I did this for about six weeks. Now as you can imagine, this wasn't the most socially acceptable thing to do, but I really felt pretty good on it until one day a blood clot got caught in my throat. That did it! That was the end of my blood-drinking days. It was good timing, as I was pretty much finished with that experiment anyway. I tell that story not to shock you, but to show you that I have tried just about everything you can imagine in attempting to experiment on myself to learn what nutritional practices work best.

I am a firm believer that what you put into your mouth has a lot to do with how you look and feel. Nutrition and exercise go hand-in-hand. You can eat perfectly, but if you don't exercise you will lose your muscle tone. On the other hand, if your diet is not perfect but if you exercise vigorously, you can get by.

I feel that I watched my father commit suicide with his knife and fork. He didn't go along with my philosophies. I'd say to him, "Dad, come exercise with me." He'd reply, "Aw, kid, that exercise is for you young kids."

My father's big hobby was shopping for food. His favorite foods were cheese, meat, and butter—primarily foods that were dairy products. He died at a very young age and I am convinced that the excessive amount of fat from the meats and cheeses contributed to his early demise.

Now my mother was just the opposite.

She was also a sickly person and had to go to a sanitarium around the time I started my gym in the backyard. When she came home she saw this tremendous change in me and wanted to learn more about nutrition. She went right along with my program of exercise and nutrition and continued until her death at the age of ninety-four. I feel that because of the change in her eating habits she added some twenty to twenty-five years to her life span. On the other hand, I feel that my Dad took about twenty-five years *off* his life because of his lifestyle and his eating habits.

Everything we do in life is a matter of habit. Habits make you what you are, make me what I am. My mother just took a few bad habits and exchanged them for good habits. Now my Dad didn't change any of his habits and look what happened to him. That was a good object lesson for me.

What all this is leading up to, I guess, is Elaine's book, *Eating Right for a New You.* She wants to give you the benefit of all the experiences, trials, and errors that we have gone through. When I first started on television in 1951, Elaine was a real junk food junkie. Besides eating badly, she smoked two packs of cigarettes a day.

She changed her eating habits, reproportioned her body, and became as enthusiastic as I am about our profession of changing the lives of people for the good. She tells her own story in the Introduction that follows.

As you read through this book, you will find that the suggestions and teachings are sensible, simple to follow, and easy to understand. They are time-proven and people-tested. My theory about life is this: What good is the Bible if you don't read it? What good is having a Rolls Royce if you never drive it? What good is this book if you never use it? The book was written to help *you* with your nutritional needs.

My mother, who as I said lived to be ninety-four, left me with these thoughts and I'd like to leave them with you:

Anything in life is possible. Make it happen!
God helps those who help themselves!
Go for it!

Introduction: Habits Our Mothers Taught Us

As the years roll along, the world in general seems to get more and more complex—and so does the world of nutrition. The storehouse of knowledge that is available to us on the subject of the foods we eat is filled to overflowing, and it is therefore confusing. No sooner is one study released saying that certain foods are good for you than another one comes out and says they are bad for you.

When I wade through masses of studies about the effects of food upon the human body in my ongoing attempt to learn the path to Peak Nutrition, I find that many of the new discoveries are what my husband, Jack, has been practicing since the 1930s and taught me well over thirty-five years ago.

Through it all, I think back to my mother, trying to see to her family's nutritional needs in a day and age when all of her knowledge came from what she learned from her own mother and from her mother's mother.

I grew up in Minneapolis, and for the early part of my life I stuck close to home. All my schooling took place near to home.

I also think back to my eating habits in those days. My breakfast consisted of cooked or dry cereal with lots of sugar and cream, or bacon and eggs with toast covered with butter and jelly, and a cup of cocoa with more sugar. When I went to school I took a lunch in the traditional brown paper bag and every day the sandwich was spread liberally with both butter and mayonnaise. Sometimes I would eat in the cafeteria and have macaroni and cheese with at least two glasses of milk. On the way home from school I would devour a couple of candy bars.

Dinner would be served by 6:00 or 6:30. Around the dinner hour I remember listening to radio shows like "Little Orphan Annie," "Jack Armstrong, the All-American Boy," and "I Love a Mystery." It was during the latter show that my father would arrive home from work. My brothers Ralph and Andy (short for Eugene) and I would set the table for dinner. We were constantly reminded to put out the bread and butter, salt and pepper, and sugar. Oh yes, and not to forget the jelly for the bread and cream for the coffee.

My mother tried to be very cognizant of what she fed us. We always had to have a vegetable, potatoes, and meat of some kind. We often had a cabbage salad, sliced tomatoes (when they were in season), and lots of carrots and sometimes rutabagas and parsnips. Whatever the menu, we always had a dessert. My Dad loved chocolate cake so we had that often. Our friends and relatives used to say, "Sib (my mother's nickname; her name was Sylvia) makes the best devil's food cake in all of Minneapolis." My Dad loved the cake but not the frosting and would cut it off and put it on his plate, so that after I finished my cake and he saw me eyeing his frosting, he would offer it to me. Needless to say, I accepted it with pleasure. If we didn't have cake we had pie. If you recall those days, cakes and pies were made with lots of butter, lard, or that substance that looks like white grease. Often we would go out later in the evening for ice cream.

As I grew older and started dating, my friends and I would often go to a movie and afterward set out for the local eatery for French fries and soft drinks. So you can see, my diet for the most part consisted of an overabundance of saturated fats.

In recalling my visits to my grandmother's home in Roland, Iowa, I remember my grandmother cooked much the same way as my mother did. So I am sure that the majority of the eating habits in our family were passed down from my grandmother.

When I went out on my own and moved to California, I found that I not only took those eating habits with me, but they deteriorated.

In the early 1940s I was swimming in the Minneapolis Aqua Follies and was in good condition. But by the time I first met Jack LaLanne in the early 1950s at the age of twenty-seven, I thought I was old . . . over the hill. I was working at the ABC-TV station in San Francisco as a Girl Friday on the "Les Malloy Show." I not only booked the show, but also appeared on it. At that time, I was the full support of my two children, so the strain of running a household and holding down a job didn't leave much time for caring about my eating or exercising habits. Consequently, I was a junk food junkie. I lived on Danish rolls and chocolate doughnuts for breakfast. For lunch: candy bars and soft drinks from the vending machines. For dinner: a hot dog or maybe a can of roast beef, a can of vegetables or fresh fruit, and my skin was beginning to show it. I thought that when you age, you just age, when you get sick, you just get sick, and when you get fat, you just get fat. I didn't realize that diet has much to do with it. I didn't understand that there is a relationship between nutrition and health.

Jack joined the TV gang at KGO-TV about a year after I did. Our mutual office was in the newsroom. Each day, Jack would come in filled with enthusiasm, talking with his director about his life-long profession, while I was down at the other end of the room smoking my cigarettes, eating my chocolate doughnut, and worrying about who I was going to get to replace a last-minute cancellation. I heard what have come to be known as LaLanneisms: "Ten seconds on the lips and a lifetime on the hips" . . . "Wear nature's girdle" . . . "The food you eat today is walking and talking tomorrow" . . . "Your waistline is your lifeline." One day while I was indulging, he said to me: "You should be eating apples and bananas and oranges. If I didn't like you, I wouldn't tell you this."

I looked up at him while puffing on my cigarette and said: "Oh yeah?"

After that, I began thinking about my life and the way I looked (my chestline was sinking into my waistline, while my legs were getting that washboard look). I really felt old.

Suddenly, I wanted to be nineteen again; maybe something really could be done! I went home that night and took off all my clothes and stood in front of a mirror and realized the awful truth about myself and decided that *something had to be done.*

Well, the end of this little story is that I started exercising every day at a class Jack conducted at noontime for a few interested people at the studio. I quit smoking, broiled everything I used to fry, cut out all white sugar and white flour products. In one month I saw the changes that had taken place in my body.

My skin became smoother and tighter. I reproportioned my body through exercise and diet. My eyesight even became more acute. I'm sure this had to do with my quitting smoking; as I understand it, smoking constricts the blood vessels in your eyes. Suddenly, I was a convert! I, too, wanted to preach the message to all who would listen. You see, I started slowing the aging process way back then. I'd hate to think of what I would look like today if I hadn't met Jack.

But you say, "It's too late for me. You can't teach an old dog new tricks." Wrong. It's never too late. Why, I have seen people in their sixties, seventies, eighties, even nineties, who have exchanged a few bad habits for good ones with tremendous results.

I am thoroughly convinced that there is an intimate relationship between what we eat and how we feel.

From talking with thousands of Americans over fifty years of age during the travels Jack and I have made over the past several decades, it is my feeling that no matter what the newspapers and magazines say about new discoveries on the effects of this or that food, most of us are still preparing foods and eating foods the same way we were taught by our mothers.

We got into the habit of eating that way, and we have never bothered to break the habit, in spite of the mounting evidence that your diet dictates your health in so many, many ways.

The purpose of this book is to present what I feel is a good, healthy way to eat. Good, nutritious food can make a person feel better, look better, have a whole new perspective on life. Bad foods can be instrumental in opening a person to illness, depression, moodiness, and general sluggishness. If you are what you eat, you don't want to be like the lard my mother used to pour down the drain that regularly clogged it up. No! You want to be as bright and perky as a fresh stalk of celery, as snappy as a freshly picked apple, as energetic as a salmon.

To feel and look better, to have stores of energy where before there was none, and to ward off illnesses that have plagued you, try changing some basic harmful eating habits and think in terms of moderation. My feeling is that it's never too late to teach an old dog new tricks. Just turn around a few detrimental eating habits and you'll find that it's possible to make an old dog into a new dog.

I've arranged this book into two sections. The first section deals with breaking old habits and installing new habits. The second section contains recipes for good, nutritious, *delicious* meals.

In the first half of the book, we'll talk about the current knowledge of how a diet affects health. We'll also talk about how good diet can help revive a person and make him or her feel better.

We'll also attempt to introduce new habits into your diet that will help you eventually override old, harmful habits.

Two concepts I repeat quite often are "Everything in moderation" and "Keep it simple."

Eating well is not at all complicated. It can be quite simple. Remember the old saying "And thinking makes it so." If we think it is complicated, it will be. Before you reach the end of the first half of this book, I hope a light bulb will go on over your head and you will say: "Why, this is all so simple and easy! Now I understand how it works. And I can make it work for me."

So without further ado, and with a heartfelt "Thank you" to our mothers who loved us so much, let's begin the book and in the process try to make our mothers proud of us, that we grew up never to stop learning what's good for us.

—ELAINE LALANNE
Morro Bay, California
October 1992

PART

I

The Secrets of Peak Nutrition

Ten Myths About the Way We Eat and Drink

MYTH #1. MILK IS GOOD FOR YOU

I was born and raised in Minnesota, the middle of one of America's most famous dairy areas. I don't think we ever had a meal that didn't include some product from a cow. For most meals we consumed perhaps a half-dozen milk products: everything from whole milk to butter, cream for our coffee to ice cream for dessert.

As Americans, most of us were raised to believe that milk was good for you from the day you were born to the day you died, that it builds strong bones and teeth—and bodies.

But pull out your dictionary and look up the word "milk."

This is what *Webster's Seventh New Collegiate Dictionary* has to say:

"milk—a fluid secreted by the mammary glands of females for the nourishment of their young."

When lecturing on nutrition, Jack makes this point about the habit of human beings drinking milk from cows:

"Approximately 70 percent of the people in the United States are allergic to milk. Man (meaning men and women) is the only animal that never weans itself from milk and is the only creature that does not live out its life span. For instance, a dog matures at two years old and lives six to seven times the age of maturity. Men and women reach maturity at the age of twenty-five. Six times 25 equals 150."

In one of his LaLanneisms, Jack makes this statement: "I'm planning on living to be 150 and I want you to stick around to find out!"

Jack continues on his theme of short-changing life expectancy and drinking milk:

"We've all been led to believe that we never outgrow our need for milk, when we actually outgrow our need for milk during the first years of our lives. Mammals suckled on their mothers' milk are weaned from it as quickly as it is practical so that they can become independent of the mother and fend for themselves. If this is so, then why should children, young adults, or fully grown adults be suckling on milk? Especially when it's from an entirely different species!"

Jack's point is a very good one. What other creature do you know that drinks the milk of another species? When you view it from that angle, it seems almost unnatural.

Now I must admit that due to my upbringing, I'm a milk lover. Nothing satisfies me more than a glass of cold milk. However, I've weaned myself from whole milk to nonfat milk. As the years go by, I am more and more amazed at the facts that are available to us about milk. I always thought that milk was our primary source of calcium. But this is not true. Some 80 percent of the inhabitants of this planet are unable to extract the calcium from milk products because they lack the LACP gene.

The LACP (lactose) gene produces an enzyme called lactase, which makes it possible to break down milk and absorb the calcium from it. If you do not have the LACP gene, the calcium is extracted more slowly from the milk and it passes right through your digestive system. The result is that people who lack the LACP gene and who have consumed milk all their lives can still have weak, brittle bones.

This reduction in ability to absorb the calcium from milk is a matter of race and nationality. For instance, if your ancestors come from Denmark there is roughly a 1 to 2 percent chance you will be unable to absorb calcium from milk; if your ancestors are from Africa there is a 30 to 90 percent chance you will not be able to absorb the calcium (depending on the tribe from which your ancestors came); if you are Jewish, your percentage rises to about 80 percent, and if you are from an Indian tribe from South America, you may have 100 percent intolerance. Typically, white Americans have a 6 to 8 percent malabsorption rate, Mexican-Americans about 55 percent, American Indians 65 to 95 percent, and African-Americans 70 to 75 percent.

Other problems that can occur in the absence of the lactase enzyme is that the milk can sometimes ferment in the intestines, causing the discomfort of gas and perhaps diarrhea. Unfortunately, while you do not receive the benefits of the calcium in the milk, you *do* absorb the fat and cholesterol that come in milk.

So, if you lack the LACP gene, you can drink a gallon of milk a day and you can still suffer from osteoporosis, simply because your body is not able to extract the calcium it needs. Research indicates that the most effective method of avoiding osteoporosis is to regularly perform weight-bearing exercises, such as walking.

It is also interesting to note that in order to homogenize milk, the fat molecules are reduced in size (through a high-speed homogenizer) until they are so small that they can pass through the walls of the intestines and into the bloodstream, where their cholesterol can add to the plaque building up on the artery walls, thereby causing or adding to arteriosclerosis. This is especially true if you are not exercising and lead a sedentary life.

And how about the vitamin D that is added to milk? Isn't that important to your health?

Yes, vitamin D certainly *is* important to your health, but your body makes its own vitamin D every time it is exposed to sunshine. And vitamin D is essential to your body assimilating calcium from the food you eat.

So, you ask, how do I get enough calcium to meet my daily needs? Try to get a little sunshine to build up your vitamin D, or take a vitamin A and D food supplement. Check with your doctor or nutritionist to see if you actually need additional vitamin D.

There *are* other sources of calcium besides milk. Foods rich in calcium include beans, broccoli, wheat, sunflower seeds, nuts, almonds, green peas, and soya flour.

If you are like me and still feel you *must* have milk, gradually wean yourself from whole milk (which contains 3.5 percent fat) to low-fat milk (which contains 2 percent fat), and then from low-fat milk to nonfat milk (0.5 percent fat). If you want nonfat milk to taste more like whole milk, mix in some dry nonfat milk crystals.

As far as milk and milk products are concerned, be aware of the amount of whole milk products you are consuming. Read labels. Our philosophy is "Everything in moderation." While one apple is good for you, you wouldn't eat a hundred apples a day, would you? A little milk is not going to hurt you, but it's the over-consumption of the product that can take its toll in excessive fat and cholesterol in the diet. Remember that whenever you overindulge in anything, there is a tariff to be paid.

 RECOMMENDATIONS

1. Quit whole milk "cold turkey," a method that works for many people who demand instant results—and who have tremendous will power.
2. Gradually wean yourself away by changing from whole milk (3.5 percent fat) to low-fat milk (2 percent fat) to 99 percent fat-free milk (1 percent fat) to skim milk (0.5 percent fat).
3. Take a compromise position by weaning yourself down to 99 percent fat-free milk. The milk still tastes pretty much like whole milk, and you will cut your fat consumption from milk to less than one third! To make the milk creamier, add nonfat milk powder to the 99 percent fat-free milk.
4. Also wean yourself from other products made from milk, including evaporated milk, cream, sour cream, ice cream, cheese, and butter. There are, however, quite a few fat-reduced cheeses, sour creams, etc., sold today.

MYTH #2. ALL OIL IS THE SAME

There is such a range of foods that are prepared with vegetable oils that I'm almost at a loss as to where to start.

Baked goods contain oils. Salad dressings contain oil. Spaghetti sauce contains oil. TV dinners contain oils. Potato chips contain oil. And certainly, any fried or deep-fried foods contain oil.

What is the problem with oils? Well, primarily the problem centers on their fat content.

The body needs a certain amount of fat, but Americans typically get way too much fat. No more than 30 percent of your daily food intake should consist of fat. I try to keep it around 20 to 25 percent. But even those who watch what they eat may take in more fat in a day than they realize because fats are used as an ingredient in foods that don't exactly advertise their fat content.

Fats from vegetable oils are further confusing because different kinds of fats have different effects on the human body. Every vegetable oil contains all three types of fat, but in vastly different proportions. Let's take a moment to discuss the three types of fat:

Polyunsaturates: This group is harmless and in fact can have beneficial side effects. It includes safflower oil, soybean oil, corn oil, cottonseed oil, sesame oil, sunflower oils, and most margarines. Polyunsaturate oils can be beneficial in a diet because they have the capacity to lower a person's cholesterol level. But you should still keep total calories from fat at less than 30 percent.

Monounsaturates: This group is also "safe," and includes olive oil, canola (rapeseed) oil, and peanut oils.

Saturates: This group is the troublesome one, and includes coconut oil, palm kernel and palm oils, hydrogenated oils, and outside the realm of vegetable oils includes whole milk dairy products, butter, lard, and other animal products.

The whole subject of oils and fats and cholesterol becomes confusing to some people because they tend to associate oils and fats and cholesterol as though they are the same things.

Vegetable oils *contain no cholesterol,* not even those that are high in saturated fats.

"But that doesn't make any sense," you say. "I've heard that I should avoid saturated fats because they'll increase my cholesterol, which is very bad for me."

What you heard is true.

Here's how it works.

Cholesterol, as you probably already know, is the waxy substance that collects on the artery walls and constricts the flow of blood through the arteries. Cholesterol comes only from two places: from animal-based foods and from our own bodies. (Our own bodies produce a certain amount of cholesterol in the liver because a certain amount of cholesterol is necessary to maintain life.)

Our bodies are constantly at work attempting to balance within themselves the essential elements we need to survive. Our bodies are constantly getting rid of cholesterol, while attempting to balance our bodies' needs with the supply they have onboard. Here's where the saturated fats come in:

Saturated fats interfere with the body's ability to remove cholesterol from the blood and get rid of it. Saturated fats disrupt the process of cleaning excess cholesterol from the bloodstream. So although saturated fats *contain no cholesterol themselves,* they tell the body what to do to the cholesterol that is already there, and what it tells the body is to keep the cholesterol.

So, as you can see, there are some oils out there you want to avoid. Most products have their ingredients listed on the package. If you read the ingredients on, let's say, a package of snack food, and among those ingredients are hydrogenated oils, coconut oils, or palm oils, look for another snack. And if oil is used in the preparation of the food, make certain the oil is polyunsaturated.

Fortunately, with the increasing awareness of cholesterol and the damage it can do to our arteries and subsequently to our hearts, many major companies have begun changing the oils used in their products. For instance, a number of very large snack food companies several years ago voluntarily stopped using coconut and palm oils and hydrogenated oils in the preparation of their snack foods. Other companies have not yet followed suit, so it is to your benefit to read the labels closely.

For years I could not eat a baked potato without butter—and lots of it. Or if the restaurant served hot French bread, it just didn't taste good without butter.

Well, as time went by and I learned more about cholesterol forming on my artery walls, I would think back to my early years in Minneapolis. My mother's sink would get clogged from so much grease being poured down it from the fat residue from the meats and butter and other saturated fats. I thought about my arteries clogging up and I gradually weaned myself from butter. How? Well, I used a little avocado as a spread for toast. Or I spread a little unsaturated oil on toast with a little vegetable seasoning sprinkled on top. For garlic bread, sprinkle with garlic powder.

You might ask why I didn't use margarine. Although margarine has no cholesterol, it still has fat and it still hardens at room temperature. I figured that if it hardens at room temperature, it must harden in my arteries, too. I now eat my bread and my baked potatoes without butter or margarine and have learned to enjoy them this way. Sometimes I use olive or canola oil mixed with minced garlic.

You'll recall that I mentioned earlier that all vegetable oils contain all three kinds of fats (polyunsaturates, monounsaturates, and saturates), but that the key to whether they are good or bad for you lies in their proportions of the three fats. I've listed a breakdown of the three fats below so you can understand what I mean by their relative proportions of good and bad fats. In the following chart, the numbers used refer to grams of fat per one tablespoon:

	Saturated	Mono-unsaturated	Poly-unsaturated
Corn oil	1.7	3.3	7.8
Olive	1.9	9.7	1.1
Coconut oil	12.1	0.8	0.3

As you can see, coconut oil contains plenty of saturated fats and almost no monounsaturates or polyunsaturates, while both corn oil (considered a polyunsaturated) and olive oil (a monounsaturated) contain very little saturated fat.

This plainly illustrates how oils are not all created equal, and how you can easily improve your diet (and your health) by being careful which oil you make your oil of choice.

 ## RECOMMENDATIONS

1. Instead of spreading butter or margarine on toast, lightly spread on some good vegetable oil and vegetable seasoning. Add garlic powder for garlic bread.
2. Use these good oils: canola oil, safflower oil, sunflower oil, corn oil, and soybean oil.
3. Avoid these oils: coconut oil and palm oil.

MYTH #3. COOKING IMPROVES FOOD

Do you remember the big headlines when President Bush refused to eat his broccoli on Air Force One? He claimed that he did not like broccoli and that his mother had always made him eat it. Now that he was President of the United States, he was going to refuse to eat broccoli. And, in fact, he was going to go so far as to have it banished from all meals served on Air Force One as long as he was President.

Perhaps George Bush doesn't like broccoli because his mother overcooked it. I feel that overcooking has turned off many children *and* adults to vegetables. I remember as a child, my mother would cover the vegetables with water and boil them until they were limp and mushy, pour the water down the sink, and add butter, salt, and pepper to make them taste better. Jack loved to tease my mother about her healthy sink. "Sylvia," he'd say, "you must have the healthiest sink in all of Minneapolis, with all those nutrients being poured down it."

It wasn't until I met Jack that I learned to steam my vegetables only to the edge of crunchiness. I didn't realize vegetables could taste so good without butter and salt. Jack explained to me that all vegetables contain natural salts if you don't cook them too much. I have been cooking this way since 1953.

Unless you are from an Asian family or from a family that had a very enlightened parent in charge when it came to food preparation, most people in the United States have lived most of their lives on overcooked food. Cooking habits are often passed down from one generation to the next.

The habit of overcooking food does two things, both of them bad:

1. It cooks away the essential nutrients.
2. It changes the look and consistency of the food.

Fresh crisp vegetables are filled with vitamins, minerals, and essential nutrients. But as soon as you cover them with water and begin boiling them, the water begins to leach out the nutrients and the water you pour down the sink contains the nutrients that should be going into your body.

Unless you are going to use vegetables in a salad, they certainly can use *some* cooking, so what's the best way to cook them? There are several ways. You can use a steamer. This is a little expandable gadget that fits into your pot and holds the vegetables above the water line while trapped steam works on the vegetables.

Or, you can stir-fry vegetables in Teflon-coated or variously coated frying pans with a little water or polyunsaturated oil.

I have stainless steel pots and pans and I will often put a little water in the bottom, just enough for steaming, and will bring the water to a boil while the pot is covered, then lower the heat and allow the vegetables to steam until crunchy.

(If I want my vegetables to taste as though they have butter on them, I use a small amount of polyunsaturated oil along with a vegetable seasoning and garlic powder.)

What advantage does this method have over cooking vegetables to death?

1. It preserves the taste of the vegetables.
2. It preserves the nutrients.

3. It gets you out of the kitchen faster. (Why cook for hours and then serve food you've cooked into nutritionless husks of their former selves?)

When I look back at the way people used to cook the goodness out of food, I can sort of understand it. Fifty or a hundred years ago, fresh food was not kept chilled and as fresh as it is now, and sometimes it took days and weeks for it to get to market. Also, there were no safeguards available as there are today to keep food from spoiling. If you loved your family in those days, you wanted to make certain you had cooked any germs or impurities out of the food you were serving. But today, with the availability of fresh foods and with the appliances to keep them fresh, this overcooking is unnecessary.

How about cooking meat and fish, you might wonder.

A similar philosophy applies.

Don't overcook.

Most fish (especially if it is filleted) can be prepared in just a few minutes. Fish that is thicker or more dense will take a bit longer, but fish can be baked, broiled, or poached fairly quickly. You never want to overcook fish because overcooking turns it into something that resembles shoe leather, which is probably why most people think they don't like fish.

As far as poultry goes, it should be baked slowly so that the natural juices are held in and so that the bird is cooked through. Don't undercook fowl.

And meat? Certain meats, especially pork, should be thoroughly cooked, but not overcooked. Most red meat should be served medium or even medium-rare. When you take a beautiful steak and cook it until it's well-done, you cook many of the nutrients out of it and it will never be as tender as it will be if it is served medium or medium-rare.

The conclusion I've come to is that America would be a much healthier place if Americans undercooked most of their their foods more often—they would preserve two or more times the nutrients.

Put the nutrients from your foods into your body, not down the drain as my mother used to do. Simplify your way of cooking and eating. In the process, you'll save time in which you can do other things with all that spare time you save. Cut down your cooking time and multiply your available nutrients.

Cook, but don't kill.

 RECOMMENDATIONS

1. Undercook vegetables in order to retain vitamins and minerals.
2. Substitute stir-frying for traditional frying methods.
3. Don't overcook fish or beef, but thoroughly cook fowl and pork.
4. Whenever possible, eat vegetables in their natural state: raw.

MYTH #4. FRIED FOODS ARE NOT AS HARMFUL AS YOU THINK

Jack LaLanne has a LaLanneism that goes something like this:

"God created an abundance of wonderful food on this planet, and the devil came along and invented the frying pan."

Frying food, unless it is stir-frying, is not conducive to good health.

It is initially unhealthy because when you fry, you have to use something in which to fry, and that's typically oil of some kind, which adds to the calories (and possibly the cholesterol) for that meal. (Unfortunately, some people have traditionally melted lard in the frying pan to begin the frying process, and lard is Villain Number 1 when it comes to cholesterol overload!)

Plus the fact that when you fry meat, you are sizzling it in its own juices as well as in the oils you use. Consequently, the meat absorbs and reabsorbs its own cholesterol-filled juices.

Have you seen those fast food advertisements where the workers fry hamburgers on a grill, the burgers absorbing and reabsorbing the cholesterol-filled fat juices that are fried out of them? If you insist on having a burger, you're better off going to a fast-food place where they use a moving grill, and where the juices (fat) that are burned out of the meat fall through the grill and are no longer a part of the meat.

You recall that I mentioned earlier how we had the healthiest kitchen sink drain in the state of Minnesota because my mother poured the water containing all the nutrients from the vegetables down the sink.

Well, the poor drain had a Jekyll and Hyde personality, because those nutrients from the vegetables were countered by the liquefied fat Mother would drain off the meat and pour down the sink.

If you want a dramatic example of this process, the next time you fry something, don't pour out the fat, but set the frying pan on a hotpad beside the sink and allow it to cool. What happens to it? As the temperature drops, the liquid turns to a waxy mess that desperately clings to anything and that won't budge unless you use lots of hot water and detergent to break it up. That's what happens inside your arteries.

I also remember that people back in my childhood used to save the bacon and fat drippings. They would pour the drippings into a Mason or a Bell jar and let them cool and harden to be reused instead of buying lard. When I think about that practice today, knowing what I've learned about how different foods act upon the human body, I can't help but cringe and wonder what my arteries would look like today if I had continued to eat the way I did then.

"But," you ask, "what can I do as a substitute for frying my meats and poultry?"

My favorite solution is to stir-fry in a wok. (I often use my stainless steel frying pan as a wok.) Instead of frying meat or chicken for a long time, trim off the visible fat from the meat and poultry, then cut it into small, bite-size pieces. After you get the wok or frying pan very hot with a thin film of a polyunsaturated oil (corn oil or safflower oil, for example), drop in the pieces of meat or poultry and stir them constantly, so that they cook very quickly, then drop in the vegetables. *Voilà!* You've got a quick, delicious meal that still retains its nutrients, and for those who find it a bother to cut and recut food, this method serves it in bite-size pieces.

It is because of eating plenty of fish and because of stir-frying their meals that

Asian people living in the Orient have such a low rate of heart disease. (I mention "Asians living in the Orient" because many Asians living in the industrialized nations have picked up our eating habits and are no longer immune to heart disease the way their ancestors were.)

So take a giant step toward eating in a healthier manner, use your frying pan to stir-fry only or try using a wok. Train yourself to think "broil, bake, and simmer."

 RECOMMENDATIONS

1. Except for stir-frying, try to banish the concept of frying foods from your life.
2. Instead of frying chicken, bake or roast it. Place the chicken on a metal rack above a catch-pan so that the excess fat that is cooked out of the chicken can be captured and disposed of. Remove skin before eating.
3. If you *must* eat bacon, a major cholesterol offender, bake the strips on a rack above a catch-pan, so that the excess fat drops away and is not reabsorbed.
4. Steaks, roasts? Same method.

MYTH #5. WE NEED THREE MEALS A DAY

The practice of eating three meals a day is a tradition that has been handed down from generation to generation. But the habit does not have to be cut and dried. There is no evidence that the human being *must* eat three meals a day. Some people manage quite well on one meal a day, some on two meals, and others on four, five, and even six meals. The number of meals we eat each day comes down to tradition and sometimes ethnic or cultural influences.

Most people in the world do not eat three meals a day, either because they do not have enough food or because three meals a day is felt to be unnecessary.

On the other hand, in some countries the people traditionally eat as often as six times a day, but they do not eat as much at one sitting as we do.

The importance of eating meals is to get a balance of the right amount of protein, fats, carbohydrates, vitamins, and minerals. So it is not so important *when* you get what you need, just so you *do* get what your body needs.

Certainly some people (especially diabetics who are attempting to control their disease with proper diet manipulation) need to eat religiously at certain times, or they face grave health problems.

For most of us, though, our health is not the factor that determines when we eat or how often.

I know that I was very much like Pavlov's dog during several periods of my life. The period that especially stands out in my mind was back in the 1950s when I was working in television in San Francisco.

Just like clockwork, every morning I would pass by a little doughnut shop. Unfortunately, I didn't just "pass by." I made a point of walking inside to buy several chocolate doughnuts or some bear claw Danish. I'd eat at least two right on the spot and take two or three more with me along to work. When lunchtime rolled around, I told myself I didn't have time to eat lunch so a little bell would seem to ring in my head. It would signal that I should get up and go to the vending machines and get a candy bar and a soft drink. I told myself that by doing that, I would keep my energy level up.

Occasionally I went out with some of my colleagues for a spaghetti and meatball lunch.

We are capable of programming ourselves to do just about anything we want. When I learned more about food and exercise and what it could do for me, I started to reprogram myself—to rewire the bell inside my head so that it didn't ring on cue.

When it comes to meals, I feel that breakfast is a very important meal.

Break the word "breakfast" down and what do you have? Break (the) fast. Breakfast is intended to break your overnight fasting from food. A reasonable, healthy breakfast can have a profound effect on how well your day goes. On the other hand, a typical American breakfast such as ham and eggs, bacon and eggs, and sausage and eggs with buttered toast and jelly is high in everything you don't need, and besides depositing unnecessary calories and cholesterol in your body, and fat in the spaces between your muscle tissue, it sits like a lead weight in your stomach for hours.

Proper balance of your daily intake of food is essential. My idea of a balanced breakfast would be: three or four egg whites, scrambled or coddled, a little cereal (whole grain), and a piece of fruit. What do we use on our cereal? Apple juice. Apple juice is sweet and you'd be surprised how delicious it tastes on cereal.

Remember when you do eat a meal that the benefits you derive from it don't come until several hours later. For instance, proteins take six to eight hours to digest, whereas carbohydrates take two to four hours.

We human beings are omnivorous, which means we can exist on a mixed diet. It is important when you are eating carbohydrate-rich meals, such as grains, potatoes, legumes, that you chew them very well. The chewing activates the salivary glands, and when your saliva mixes with the carbohydrates, it initiates the digestion process. It's the saliva that helps turn the starch into sugar so our body can use it. If you just gulp your food down and do not salivate, the digestion of the starches is inhibited. You cannot metabolize and utilize your starchy foods unless they are broken down into usable sugars, which in turn provide energy.

While we're on the subject of carbohydrates and myths, many people seem to think that whole grains have fewer calories than processed white grains. Not so. The grains are all the same. But the whole grains have a bonus: they also have fiber and additional vitamins and minerals.

How are proteins digested? When you eat meat or any type of protein (beans, for instance), the hydrochloric acid in your stomach works to digest the protein. So instead of your salivary glands doing the work, your stomach undertakes the task.

Some people are finding that it is much easier on their stomachs if they "graze" instead of eating regular meals. What this means is that instead of eating three regular meals a day, they eat perhaps five or six times, but in much smaller portions. If you graze rather than eat regular meals, you must remember to be certain you receive a balanced diet.

"Grazing" is entirely different from "snacking."

When I think of snacking, I always think of my dear aunt who was famous to all her friends and neighbors and relatives for her angel food cakes. She loved her coffee and cigarettes and picked and snacked a lot. When I would ask her about her little snacks, she would say, "Oh, this is hardly anything." But lots of "hardly anythings" add up to a lot of something. She was overweight, had heart trouble (the painful kind, angina), but never considered that her eating habits may have had something to do with her weight and her angina.

I could not convince her that picking and snacking added up to many more calories than if she had had only three meals a day.

On the flip side of the coin, many people will starve themselves all day and wait until the evening meal to eat, with perhaps a few little snacks in between to keep them going. Then at dinner they will overindulge because they are so hungry. They end up consuming more calories than they would have had they eaten three meals. Then they wonder why they can't lose weight. After all, they eat only one meal a day.

Then there are those who just don't like to cook for themselves. These are typically people who live alone. They never seem to be hungry and end up starving themselves to death.

The number of meals you have a day is not the important thing. What is important is the balance in your diet and the quality of the foods you eat.

What you ingest is calculated by using calories. For instance, if you need 1,500 calories a day to maintain your weight and you eat 1,000, you are going to lose weight. If you eat 2,000 calories, you are going to gain weight. Each of us should calculate how many calories a day we need to maintain ourselves, and we should make certain that the calories we consume are not hollow calories. The calories need to be in the proper proportion from proteins, carbohydrates, and fats, and they need to bring adequate vitamins and minerals and roughage along with them. The highest octane calories we can eat come from natural foods in their natural state.

The slavish adherence to eating three meals every day, and perhaps having one or two snacks along the way, is a habit that is certainly unnecessary as we age. Our metabolisms slow down and our bodies do not need food as often or in the quantities as when we were eighteen years old. Even the fifty-plus person who is exercising does not need as much food/fuel as the comparable eighteen-year-old.

If you aren't hungry, it is your body's way of saying it doesn't need food at the moment. If your body isn't hungry, don't feed it just because it's noon and therefore it's lunchtime.

Listen to your body. You'll be surprised what it will tell you.

 RECOMMENDATIONS

1. Eat an adequate, nutritious breakfast. Breakfast is the most important meal of the day.
2. Don't eat if you aren't hungry.
3. Don't snack and eat between meals.
4. Don't take in more calories than you're burning up.
5. Don't starve yourself. Eat enough each day to provide a balanced diet.

MYTH #6. ALL MEAT IS BAD FOR YOU

Everywhere you turn, there is new information on what you should and should not eat. To further complicate matters, one study will recommend eating one particular food and the next study will recommend that you not eat it.

It was so much easier when we were young and we were taught just to eat what our mothers put in front of us. As we know today, though, blindly eating what is put in front of us is not very good for our health.

It is important to have a store of current knowledge of which foods are good for us and which are not. As we discussed in Myth #2, all oil is not the same, and it can add years to your life to know which is which.

Likewise, it is to your benefit to have a good knowledge of what is safe to eat and what is not in virtually every category of food.

Perhaps the area of food that has come in for the most confusing claims over the last decade is meat.

We underwent a barrage of claims about the dangers from meat in the wake of hearing about the dangers from high cholesterol.

Animal meats contain fat. The fat in animal meats is high in cholesterol, but the primary problem is that it is saturated fat.

Generally, we have been raised to think of "meat" as being beef, pork/ham, veal, lamb, and game such as deer and rabbit. In the strict dietary sense, however, animal meat also includes poultry (turkey, chicken, duck, game hen, etc.) and fish (including crustaceans such as lobster and shellfish).

Because of the size and resources of our country, and because of more efficient methods of raising them, animal meats such as beef and pork and lamb have been more affordable than they are in most countries in the world. Therefore, it has been almost un-American to serve a major meal *without* some sort of meat, whether it be the Sunday chuck roast or the July 4th chicken barbecue.

Animal meat has long been America's favorite source of protein.

Unfortunately, protein from animals cannot be separated from cholesterol in animal fats.

Fortunately, there are some relatively easy guidelines that can be applied that will allow you to substitute good meat for bad meat.

Let's take a moment to look at some very simple guidelines that will allow you to continue serving meat at your meals without having to worry that "all meat is bad."

Serve meat less often. Many people feel they must serve some sort of meat at every meal of the day. I know my mother felt that way. This is not necessarily true. There are other dietary sources of protein, such as beans, that come without the accompanying undesirable fat and cholesterol. Why not attempt to cut back to serving meat at only *one* meal a day instead of at all three?

Serve smaller portions of meat. You can save a great deal of money on your grocery bill over a week's time if you cut back the amount of meat you buy. Instead of buying large portions of meat products, attempt to be more selective: go for a smaller, leaner cut, and you'll get the same amount of protein without the accompanying fats and cholesterol.

Trim off fat. This applies to any type of meat, from pork to chicken. Trim off any excess fat you find on the meat you buy. On a steak or roast, trim away the excess fat around the edge of the meat. Some supermarkets are now offering meats that are more closely trimmed.

Soy-based meat extenders or beans can also be used to reduce your total consumption of meat.

Pick cuts that are more lean. Cattle ranchers are now raising more lean beef, and many supermarkets are offering leaner grades of beef in response to the consumers' demands for beef that will not raise their cholesterol.

Remove chicken and turkey skin. Both chicken and turkey can be made even less harmful in the high-cholesterol battle if, before you prepare them, you remove the skin. Or, if you prepare the chicken or turkey with the skin, cook it on a rack above a catch-pan so that most of the fat drips off. *Then,* before you serve it, remove the skin. In poultry, dark meat contains about twice the fat and cholesterol as white meat.

Learn which meat products are high in cholesterol and which are low. Here is a chart to give you an example of this:

	High cholesterol	*Low cholesterol*
Beef	sirloin	rump
Pork	Canadian bacon	center-cut ham
Veal	breast	most other cuts*
Lamb	loin	leg of lamb
Chicken	large hens	Cornish game hen
Fish	salmon	cod
Shellfish	lobster	shrimp
Game	————	most game is lean

*The above listings are *relative* to the type of meat mentioned. For instance, veal is higher in cholesterol than beef or pork, but in picking cuts of veal, the breast of veal is higher in cholesterol than other cuts.

By doing a little research on meat, it becomes quite clear that not all meat is created equal. So, to answer the question: "Is all meat bad for you?" The answer is a resounding "No!" Learn your meats. There are charts available from a variety of sources that will give you guidelines for which cuts of meat are leaner and lower in cholesterol. In fact, many meat counters at the local supermarkets feature such charts. Do a little research into meat before you buy your cuts, and go for the lean!

What follows is a list of meat products to avoid because of their *high fat and cholesterol* content:

Beef: T-bone, sirloin, rib (small end), porterhouse, any fatty cut.

Pork: There are no lean cuts of pork, but the leanest in a non-lean category are center-cut ham, sliced ham, pork tenderloin, and loin chops.

Veal: The breast, although as we mentioned above, veal is more cholesterol-saturated than its beef and pork counterparts.

Lamb: Rib chops, lamb shank, loin.

Poultry: Older and larger birds are higher in fat.

Fish: Although some fish are fattier than others, all fish is good for you due to its omega-3 oil, which has been shown to reduce cholesterol.

High-risk kinds of meat products that you should avoid:

All organ meats: Liver, kidneys, heart, sweetbreads, brains.

High fat: Bacon, ham hocks, spareribs, picnic ham, regular hamburger, brisket, tongue, duck, goose, compressed veal patties, pork butt, pigs' feet and ears.

Super high fat: Hot dogs, canned meat, sausages, luncheon meats (these products are well over 75 percent fat).

To balance this out, what are some of the best meats you can eat?

Broiled fish, tuna packed in water, white turkey meat, broiled scallops, or lean, trimmed cuts of beef, pork, or veal.

The way you prepare your meat has a profound effect upon its effect upon you. As we've mentioned before, frying or stewing meats merely recycles the fats and cholesterol you're trying to get rid of. Instead of frying or stewing, broil or roast your meat, fish, and poultry. This process allows the harmful fats to drip off the meat so you have essentially discarded them in the cooking process and much of the fat is gone from the food when you finally eat it.

 RECOMMENDATIONS

1. Trim off excess fat.
2. Broil instead of fry.
3. Cook meat so that fat drops into bottom of pan and is not reabsorbed by meat.
4. Remove poultry skin.

MYTH #7. SALT IS A SPICE

When I go to a restaurant and see a waitress bring food to a table only to have the diners automatically grab for the salt shaker to sprinkle it onto the food before they even taste it, I feel my teeth grinding together. I have to just about tie myself to my chair so I don't rush over to that person's table to talk to them about what they are doing, not only to perfectly good food, but to their bodies.

I become equally distressed when I see someone take a TV dinner out of the oven and sprinkle salt onto it. Most processed foods already have enough salt in them to turn a swimming pool into the Salton Sea.

The practice of sprinkling salt on everything that goes into a person's mouth as though it somehow enhances the food is one of the major dietary afflictions in our society.

People use salt as though it were a spice. It's not; it's a chemical.

Food packagers use salt to cover the taste of their foods and to help preserve the foods longer, to give them a longer "shelf life." I also believe our mothers used a lot of salt to cover the bland taste of vegetables overcooked in water.

Unfortunately, an overabundance of salt can have some very disastrous effects. It can cause you to retain water in your system and become bloated and it can also raise blood pressure to dangerous levels, which leads to heart disease, stroke, and kidney disease.

Salt is a mineral composed of two elements, sodium and chlorine; if we weighed a tablespoon of salt, 40 percent of its weight would come from sodium.

Now here's where the problem comes in: Nearly one out of every five Americans is a walking time bomb from a genetic standpoint in that their bodies are set to self-destruct if the fuse is lit. And guess what the fuse is. Sodium. The self-destruction comes in the form of hypertension, and the presence of hypertension causes a variety of very important body organs to fail.

I mentioned before that a person who ingests too much salt tends to become bloated. What happens is that salt pulls water to itself inside the body in an attempt to make itself more dilute, to attempt to reach a balance in the fluid that surrounds our body cells.

That's why if you eat a salty potato chip, you suddenly feel the urge to drink something. Your body wants to dilute the sodium you've just added, and your body is telling you it needs water or some other fluid to get the job done, so you become thirsty. *Now* you've eaten sodium (salt) and taken onboard more fluid, which has added to your weight, and to your feeling of bloating.

Under normal circumstances, when you have too much sodium in your body, the excess is leached out by the kidneys and dumped into the urine, where you excrete it. But if you've been forcing your kidneys to do this job constantly for years because you consistently eat too much salt, the kidneys eventually begin malfunctioning, like an overworked chemical plant, and they can no longer keep up.

Eventually, this excess sodium is trapped in the body and wants to pull more and more fluid to itself. Your blood volume is therefore increased until, in a sort of reaction to overload, the blood vessels narrow and the heart has to pump like crazy to push this excessive amount of blood through ever-smaller openings, thus creating increased pressure, hence high blood pressure. Under those circumstances, the poor heart is working itself to death—figuratively and literally.

And all because you got into the habit of eating too much salt.

Except for the strenuous exerciser and the laborer who works in hot conditions and sweats profusely, the typical American adult should not have to add salt to anything—his or her daily requirement of sodium is more than filled by the presence of sodium in regular foods and water. (And for those who *do* sweat a great deal either because of work or exercise, *do not use salt tablets*. The sodium concentration is much too high, and instead of helping your body function properly, the salt will actually draw fluids from inside your cells, where the fluid is needed, and into the surrounding fluid, where it is useless.)

Our appetite for salt is learned, not natural. There is no evidence that ancient man added salt to what he ate. He received his needed sodium from the foods he ate.

We begin our "thirst" for salt when we are infants. As we are being weaned from milk, we are being trained to tolerate the taste of salt, and then to crave it. Many studies of widely different cultures have been made, and it has been found that many cultures do not use sodium at all: they ingest only the sodium that is in the food and water they consume. And guess what? Those cultures have almost no hypertension or high blood pressure.

On the other hand, cultures that do use a lot of salt (for instance, in northern Japan) have extremely high rates of hypertension and high blood pressure—and death from heart and kidney disease.

One of the best things you can do for your body—and especially for your heart, kidneys, and blood vessels—is to drastically cut your salt intake. Certainly, like any other habit, such as smoking or drinking, salt addiction is something that you'll have to fight.

Perhaps the best way to do it is to go cold turkey. Just give it up. You might be surprised at how quickly you adapt to a saltless lifestyle. You will also be surprised at how your taste gradually comes back, and you are able to appreciate the taste of foods for what they are, instead of tasting merely the salt that hides or leaches away their taste.

There are currently a variety of salt substitutes on the market that satisfy your desire for salt, but that do not contain sodium, and they are worth trying. I find that garlic powder is a wonderful seasoning.

The greatest challenge facing someone who wants to kick the salt habit, however, is that there is so much salt put into processed or store-bought foods that it's difficult to find products that are salt-free. There is a high concentration of sodium in some foods where you wouldn't expect it, from breakfast cereals to bread, butter to canned soup.

Fortunately, in today's more health-conscious America, food companies have become convinced that there is a market out there for "low-salt" and/or "no-salt" products and they have responded with a whole array of processed foods that will help the average American get control of hypertension and high blood pressure.

The first and best step you can take is to get up right now, walk to your kitchen, find the salt shaker(s), and hide them. Then begin living a saltless lifestyle. Your heart, your kidneys, and your whole body will thank you.

And don't be surprised if you begin to lose weight (in the form of retained water) in the process.

 RECOMMENDATIONS

1. Don't salt your food until you've tasted it. It's an insult to the chef.
2. Use natural herbs and spices instead of salt.
3. Read the contents of prepared foods to detect hidden salt.
4. If you've been in the habit of using excess salt, have your blood pressure monitored on a regular basis.
5. When shopping, look for salt-free versions of the product.

MYTH #8. SUGAR IS A FOOD FOR ENERGY

I don't think I've ever met anyone who gets up on his soapbox and talks about the deleterious effects of white sugar as often as does Jack LaLanne.

He tells some harrowing stories of what he was like as a youngster when he was a sugarholic. He had uncontrollable fits of temper, he suffered from melancholy and was always depressed, his skin was covered with pimples and boils, he had suicidal tendencies, couldn't concentrate in school, and was sickly all the time. This dreadful existence grew out of his mother's addicting him to sugar by using candy to bribe him to become potty trained when he was an infant. But as soon as he kicked the sugar habit, Jack's life was turned around: his complexion improved, as did his grades in school; he no longer had an uncontrollable temper, and his general health improved greatly.

A little bit of sugar is not of itself harmful. It's overconsumption that causes the problem. As we've said before, "Moderation in all things" is a motto by which we should all live. The problem comes when we tend to overindulge. And because of the amount of sugar hidden away in so many products, we overindulge without even knowing it.

Many of us take sugar for granted. We grew up with it and it's in almost everything we eat.

So let's take a moment to dispel the myth that sugar is food.

To test the question of whether sugar is food, simply look at the four food groups: meat and fish, dairy products, grains, fruits and vegetables. Sugar is not mentioned.

In reality, sugar, just like salt, is an additive. And it's an additive that we Americans add to everything, whether we do it personally at home or at a food processing factory.

The largest problem we face with regard to sugar is its accessibility. So much of it is disguised and used in foods that we are not even aware of it. Sure, we know there's sugar in ice cream and cake frosting, in jams and jellies, and in soft drinks and candy. But there's also quite a bit of salt *and* sugar in ketchup, salad dressings, bread, canned goods, cured hams, breakfast cereals—the list goes on and on.

The most common sugar we encounter comes from sugar cane or sugar beets, and it is a disaccharide (sucrose), which is one molecule of glucose paired with a molecule of fructose. Sucrose is Jack's arch-enemy: table sugar—white, refined sugar. But the problem is not confined to table sugar; it also includes brown sugar and powdered sugar.

The FDA (Food and Drug Administration) has proposed (November 7, 1991) that the grams of sugar per serving be listed on the nutritional panel. This proposal was eligible to become law as of November 1992. Sweeteners will be grouped together on the nutritional panel to make it easier for consumers to gauge the sugar content of a product.

Sugar has no additional nutritional value because the calories in the sugar are hollow. The only thing it has is calories. Empty calories.

And please don't deceive yourself into thinking that one type of sugar is different from another, or that honey is not a sugar. All sugar is pretty much the same. Honey is a type of sugar and has the same amount of calories as white sugar. Proponents of using honey contend that it is preferable to plain sugar because it contains vitamins and minerals and other nutrients, but those substances are present in only minute quantities, and for those who are allergic to bee stings, honey that is not extensively processed can contain substances from the bees that made it that can cause allergic reactions. The more processed and overheated the honey in the preparation stages, the more like plain white sugar the sugar in the honey becomes. Before using only honey as your sweetener, it is wise to research the processing techniques used on the brand you wish to purchase. I've used honey in cooking since 1953, but I've always checked out the processing sources.

Sugar also contributes to weight problems because calories are hidden in so many processed foods and are so easy to accumulate.

Natural sugars, as they exist in fruit and sugar cane, have all the B vitamins necessary for their own assimilation by the body. Our bodies do not readily store B vitamins; it is therefore essential to maintain an ongoing supply of these important vitamins. Sugars that do not come equipped with their own supply of B vitamins make it necessary for the body to give up its stores of B vitamins in order to process and store the sugar, thereby depleting the body's store of the all-important B vitamins. Since the B vitamins in the body are important to the proper function of the nerves, muscles, kidneys, stomach, heart, and even the skin, eyes, and blood, those body systems are put at risk. Take a good look at the people around you. We are a nation of people with frayed nerves, stomach disorders, heart trouble, poor eyesight, muscular diseases, and assorted skin diseases. These maladies don't just happen by themselves.

Much more serious, however, are the potential problems from diabetes and hypoglycemia.

We still do not know exactly how diabetes works, but we know that the many people suffering from it exhibit a persistent thirst and an excessive discharge of urine. Chemically, diabetes involves a shortcoming in the pancreas's ability to pump out enough insulin when the diabetic puts food into his or her body and it is absorbed in the intestines, which raises the blood sugar.

As even the most unscientific person knows, eating sugar really shoots the blood sugar up and makes you feel good and energetic almost immediately. The pancreas reacts by sending out insulin to take excess sugar out of the blood so it can be stored safely as fat. The diabetic, however, is unable to put out enough insulin to get the sugar out of the blood. Also, the more overweight a person is, the less capable that person is of getting the sugar molecules where they belong.

Although we believe that certain people are genetically prone to developing diabetes, experiments have shown that people can become diabetic simply by eating too much sugar. Other experts blame obesity for the onset and perpetuation of diabetes.

Either way, since excessive consumption of sugar can cause one to become overweight, and since either or both excess sugar consumption and obesity are contributing factors to diabetes, it is best to address both issues by cutting down on sugar intake and by losing weight. In most cases, of course, if you cut down on sugar, you'll automatically lose some weight.

One thing that fascinates me as I listen to people following our lectures is the number of people who will tell me they are both diabetic and hypoglycemic. Hypoglycemia seems to have become an "in" disease over the past decade or so. In reality, very few people suffer from clinical hypoglycemia. And *certainly,* diabetics don't, because hypoglycemia is just the opposite of diabetes. Instead of the pancreas not being able to produce enough insulin to help the absorption of foods, the pancreas turns out *too much* insulin, which takes too many sugar molecules out of the blood, resulting in a tremendous drop in energy, faintness, and general dullness.

Any person can get an idea of what true hypoglycemia is like simply by going without food for four or five hours, then eating a candy bar. There will be an immediate sugar rush, and that will be followed by a tremendous letdown or drop in energy. But for the true hypoglycemic, you'd need to multiply this normal effect several times.

There is also some persuasive research that indicates that a high consumption of sugar can raise one's blood triglyceride levels, which in turn cause atherosclerosis, or hardening of the arteries, and consequently heart disease, this country's number one killer of adults.

As with salt, a person can stop cold turkey with sugar, and the good results become apparent in a number of days. Jack claims that when he quit eating sugar, he began to see the good results in a matter of two days.

As with salt, however, the problem is placed in perspective when you realize how much sugar is hidden away in foods. Consider breakfast cereals, for instance. Did you know that more than half of the total weight of a number of breakfast cereals comes from sugar? Read the labels and compare cereals, including granolas.

And don't let advertising mislead you into believing that if you're feeling a little low, a little tired in the afternoon, all you have to do is eat a candy bar and you'll be jet-propelled. Instead of being jet-propelled, you'll be more like a July 4th bottle rocket: There will be a short, intense surge of energy, followed by a very rapid drop-off of energy, until what little energy you have left is exploded away. Eating a candy bar (or any sugar-based food) in the hopes of getting quick energy, or a quick pick-me-up, is faulty thinking. You'll not only go up like a rocket, you'll come down like a spent rocket; in fact, when you come down, you'll come down farther than you were *before* you ate the sugar. If you eat more sugar at that point, you'll once again go up and you'll drop even farther. And at the end of it all, you'll be ready to lie down to take a nap—but you'll be taking a nap several hundred calories fatter than you were when you felt a little tired and needed a boost.

 RECOMMENDATIONS

1. Try to reduce your sugar intake.
2. Avoid candy or soft drinks that contain sugar.
3. Avoid highly sugared baked goods.
4. Avoid using sugar to sweeten your coffee or tea; use a sugar substitute.
5. Read labels and avoid processed foods that are high in sugar.
6. Don't keep a secret cache of candy around the house. You won't eat what you don't have.

MYTH #9. WE DON'T NECESSARILY NEED EIGHT GLASSES OF WATER A DAY

Although the emphasis of this book is to change generations'-old dietary habits in the interest of better fitness and health, there are some age-old pieces of advice that I heartily endorse and that I have preached for years.

One of my favorites involves the most overlooked substance the human body can ingest—water.

The age-old adage is that you should drink eight glasses of water a day if you want to foster good health.

I'll bet everyone reading this book has heard that one. And by the same token, I'll bet at least 90 percent of you have, for one reason or another, completely ignored it.

Some of you may drink less water than you should because you associate water with the body's ability to retain water, and in doing so can make you feel bloated. Some people feel they get enough water in the juices and foods they eat in a typical day. Some of you may feel it is only necessary to drink eight glasses if you are physically active. Some of you may feel that with aging your metabolism slows, and therefore you do not require the same amount of water you once did.

Life on this planet is impossible without water. Life as we know it came from the sea; human life begins in the womb, the fetus encased in a watery environment.

The body of a newborn is composed of some 85 percent water. The typical adult female is about 60 percent water, the typical adult male about 70 percent water.

Every cell in our body depends heavily on water for its existence and needs to be bathed in water in order to function properly. (Think of your body cells deprived of water as either an automobile engine running without oil or a gate opening on rusty hinges.)

Water is important as the main ingredient of our blood. It is important in the daily flushing of waste materials from our bodies, both liquid and solid. Water (through sweating, both noticeable and unnoticed) helps regulate our body temperature. Water cushions our brains inside our skulls. Water is important in the lubrication effect needed for joints to work properly. Water inside our individual cells allows those cells to function efficiently, while water that surrounds the cells prevents the individual cells from sticking together and thereby undermining their smooth functioning.

A person never outgrows a need for water.

On a daily basis, our bodies use (and lose) water in three ways:

1. Through urine.
2. Through perspiration from the skin and exhalation from the lungs.
3. Through bowel movements.

How much water do these regular body functions use each day? For the average person, roughly 90 to 100 ounces.

From what sources do our bodies receive water? Primarily from three sources:

1. A small amount comes from oxidation processes happening within the body.
2. A fair amount comes from eating solid foods, which typically contain quite a bit of water. (For instance, iceberg lettuce is 95 percent water.)
3. The rest (more than half) must come from drinking water and other liquids that contain water.

What if I told you that drinking a sufficient amount of water each day would:

Help you lose weight and keep it off
Curb your appetite
Promote regularity
Help slow aging
Promote better skin
Promote physical flexibility
Help reduce headaches

Well, drinking a sufficient amount of water each day will do all of those things. Here's how it works:

Lose weight and keep it off. "What?" you are probably saying. "But water retention adds to a person's weight." We're not talking about water retention here. (Water retention can often be prevented merely by cutting down on the amount of salt in your diet.) We're talking about drinking water to lose weight. Let's allow Dr. Richard Powell of Santa Rosa, California, to explain it. Dr. Powell specializes in bariatrics (weight loss): "The kidneys get rid of toxic metabolites in the body. They have to work overtime if they don't get enough water. If the kidneys can't handle the toxic substances, you get a high level in the blood. Then the liver has to do it and can't metabolize fat as well." Additionally, a shortage of water in the body causes production of a hormone that causes salt retention as the body attempts to keep body fluid levels at an adequate level. "If you drink enough water," Dr. Powell says, "you actually wash this excess salt out." Additionally, too little water intake can cause stones to form. "The first thing we do is set a big (half-gallon) pitcher of water in front of them (dieters) and say, 'Make sure you kill this every day.'"

Curb appetite. Sufficient intake of water on a regular basis can also curb appetite, further adding to weight loss and weight maintenance since water contains no calories, and excess water is excreted by the body, unless you do something to retain it. "Water also suppresses appetite, keeps the stomach full to some extent," Dr. Powell says, thereby restricting calorie intake.

Regularity. An incredible number of older Americans, especially women, complain about the problems of irregularity. They go to doctors for the problem and they consume enormous amounts of laxatives, which, taken *too* frequently, can actually *cause* additional irregularity. One of the primary causes of irregularity is lack of sufficient water in the stool to allow the fecal matter to move through the bowels quickly and efficiently. By increasing your daily intake of water and eating sufficient fiber each day, you will be surprised at how regularity returns. (Of course, an additional way to promote regularity is to exercise aerobically on a regular basis.) And keep in mind that regularity is an important deterrent to cancer; fecal matter that sits for days in the bowels has been proven to promote the chances of cancer.

Helps slow aging. The body is made up of billions of individual cells that work together to function as a complex organism. Each cell has a life of its own. Cells that are regularly deprived of necessary fluid begin to dry up and age at a tremendous rate. Keep the cells bathed in fluid and they'll function better, longer, and will stay young and efficient.

Better skin. The human skin is composed of millions of specialized cells. Dry the cells out with too much sun or too much dehydration, and the skin becomes stiff, leathery, and old. Consume sufficient water and you assist your skin in staying supple and healthy.

Physical flexibility. As we age we get stiff in the joints for two reasons: lack of exercise and drying out of the specialized tissues. The joints and ligaments need to be properly hydrated in order to remain limber and flexible. Dry them out and, like a tree deprived of water, they become stiff and brittle—and they crack at the first strong wind.

Helps reduce headaches. The brain is encased in a reservoir of fluid that keeps it from bumping against the inside of the skull. If you are low on fluids, the amount of fluid available to cushion the brain decreases and the brain becomes susceptible to irritated nerve endings, which can cause severe headaches. (This is one of the reasons for hangovers: Someone who overimbibes alcohol depletes the fluid cushioning the brain inside the skull because alcohol has a dehydrating effect. Any process of dehydration causes the fluids in all parts of the body to drop, and when it drops inside the skull, it can cause painful headaches.)

So what are the guidelines for drinking sufficient water?

Drink eight eight-ounce glasses of water a day. The water doesn't have to all be in the form of plain water. It can come in the form of fruit juices (although then you are taking in extra calories) or diet soft drinks. You do not have to drink all eight glasses at once. Keep a water bottle around and *sip* water all day. You don't have to guzzle it down.

Remember that the sensation of thirst comes on once you are already well on the road to dehydration. Don't wait until you become thirsty to drink.

A good gauge of proper hydration is your urine. If it is yellow or golden, very concentrated, you are behind in your fluids. Your urine should be clear and you should urinate regularly throughout the day.

Next time you think in terms of your overall health, raise a glass of water, and say to yourself, "I'll drink to that!"

 RECOMMENDATIONS

1. Drink at least eight glasses of water a day.
2. Add freshly squeezed lemon to water to make it more palatable.
3. Buy a squeeze bottle so you can carry your water with you.
4. Substitute flavored mineral waters for soft drinks.

MYTH #10. ALL FLOURS ARE ALIKE

When Jack was a youngster, he faced a very unfortunate and distressing life due in large part to living under the dictates of a very bad diet. In Myth #8, I told you about the problems he had with sugar and sugar products, how it warped his personality, caused him to be sick frequently, and generally messed up his life. Jack is one of the kindest, most caring people I know, and he wouldn't hurt a fly, but to this day, when the subject of refined sugar comes up, his blood rises, his voice rises, and it is filled with passion. If there were a sugar beet around, I have the feeling he'd begin jumping up and down on it.

Although he saves sugar for Public Enemy Number 1, he is nearly as passionate about white flour.

In fact, during his first day on TV in 1951, Jack was so enthusiastic that he wanted to change everyone's life—he wanted them to eat better and exercise more. He used audio-visual aids to illustrate his point on the perils of eating white bread. He took a loaf of white bread, complete with manufacturer's wrapper, showed it to his television audience, and went on and on about how this long loaf of white bread had no nutritional value and was filled with empty calories. He took the bread out of the wrapper and put it between his two hands, then rolled it up into a ball and threw it on the floor, where it made a big thud.

Jack exclaimed: "Bang! That's what it does when it hits your stomach—and then your stomach has to work overtime to digest it."

Well, needless to say, no sooner had he mentioned all this than the bread company was on the phone, saying, "Get that crackpot off the air or we'll withdraw all our advertising from your station!"

You can bet that Jack never showed a label again when he was trying to make a point.

The company didn't take its advertising off the air, and eventually it even came out with a whole grain bread.

Jack's complaint, and my complaint about white flour and the products that are made from them, is that the life forces have been taken from them. Take the wheat kernel, for instance. Of itself, it is a perfectly balanced food. It supplies things our body requires. Unfortunately, in so many of the white flour products found on the grocery shelves, we don't get everything that was in the whole kernel at the outset.

Modern milling and processing methods have robbed the grains of their very life forces. Chemicals have to be added to prevent mold and the flour has been bleached to make it appear white. Artificial vitamins have been put back into the flour, enriching the bread, when the whole kernel was enriched to start with.

It is easiest to picture a grain of wheat by thinking of something we are more familiar with: an egg, but an egg with a very, very small yolk.

The outer shell is called the bran. The bran is like the clothes that protect the insides from the elements. There are about a half-dozen layers of bran around a grain or kernel of wheat, protecting the insides just as the shell of an egg protects what's inside. The bran has no calories, and when you eat it, it merely passes through your system, cleaning out your intestines as it goes. This is why people need bran in their diet—because it is fiber. Although the bran does not contain calories, it does contain a wonderful array of B vitamins, which the intestines can extract while the bran is passing through doing its job, cleaning the intestines, and in making people regular. When the grain is milled, the bran is removed and so are the B vitamins and the cleansing properties.

Next, there is the germ. This would be comparable in the egg to a miniature yolk. The germ is the part of the grain that allows it to serve as a seed, to sprout and make more wheat or oat or rice. The germ contains some vegetable oil (the good kind), vitamin E, and many B vitamins similar to those contained in the bran. Between the bran and the germ, they also contain 27 percent of the total protein of the grain. When it is milled, all those good things go by the wayside and the little bit of vegetable oil contained in the germ is extracted in order to increase shelf life.

What do we have left? We have the endosperm, or what is comparable to the white of the egg. The endosperm constitutes about 75 percent of the kernel of wheat. It is mostly starch, although it does contain good portions of the B vitamins, riboflavin and pantothenic acid.

By the time the endosperm gets to the other end of the milling process, it has lost about 80 percent of the nutrients that the grain originally had, it contains less than one fourth of the original vitamin E, and nearly all of the fiber content has been stripped away by removal of the bran. As if that's not bad enough, what's left is then bleached, a process that destroys even more of the vitamin E.

The way the mill attempts to overcome this wholesale destruction of the good of the grain is by artificially putting back some of the vitamins and minerals. That's what the word "enriched" on the package of flour means.

The flour you get when you buy white, enriched flour is a mere shadow of the wonderfully nutritious grain that began the process in the mill. So your basic white bread is pretty much what it feels like when you hold a slice in your hand: nothing.

What kind of flour should you use if you bake? I use stone-ground whole grain flour. In baking for instance, I use whole wheat pastry flour. Give it a try.

If you're buying bread, buy bread made with stone-ground flour or with whole wheat or whole grain of some kind. Just because a bread is brown or a darker color doesn't mean it's made with whole grain. Read the label.

It's to your advantage not to be living in a white bread world. Be adventurous. Live a little. In fact, live a lot. Go for the whole kernel. Believe me, you'll be healthier for it!

 RECOMMENDATIONS

1. Avoid bleached flour.
2. Use whole grain flour.

How Your Diet and Lifestyle Habits Can Affect Your Health

Some years ago I heard of a very interesting remedy for a recurring back problem that had for decades bothered a male friend of ours. Our friend had suffered from chronic lower back problems for nearly thirty years. He had been to one doctor after another and had undergone some costly and painful therapy.

One day, as fate would have it, he was at his daughter's house, two thousand miles from home, and his back began acting up again. His daughter quickly made an appointment for him to be seen by a doctor she knew. The doctor examined our friend, found him to be generally in good health, and also found that his back was relatively stable and in good condition. "In which of your back pockets do you carry your wallet?" the doctor asked our friend.

"Why, in the right pocket," he answered.

"Try carrying it in your suit jacket," the doctor said.

Our friend never had a back problem after that.

From spending years and years sitting at a desk with his wallet in his right rear pocket, the wallet had acted like a wedge and had thrown off this man's spine, just as a car can have a front end alignment problem that will wear down tires unevenly. With the wallet removed, our friend was a new man, his back was back to normal.

I tell this story because, having been around for more than a few years, and having seen people in all levels of fitness and health—from sixty-year-olds who can run a marathon in less than four hours to fifty-year-olds who can't get from one side of the room to the other—I've found that many health problems that seem chronic and insurmountable are often susceptible to the simple removal of one thing or the addition of something else. And this removal or addition often involves the diet.

Are you chronically constipated?

Take a long, hard look at your daily intake of fiber, your water consumption, and your level of exercise. In almost every instance I've ever encountered, the constipation can be helped by changing from a breakfast high in fats, cholesterol, and meats that tend to stay in the intestines for a very long time, and that are not easily digested, to a breakfast of hot cereal high in bran covered with nonfat milk or apple juice, some fresh fruit, and followed by a one-mile walk.

I'd like to use this chapter to look at a variety of diseases only too common to the American public (and especially to the more mature American), and then consider what foods can be eliminated from the diet or added to your way of life that will have a positive influence.

Now, let's take time to look at a series of eight health problems or diseases that are common among Americans over fifty, and let's examine how diet affects them:

CANCER

If there is one thing I find distressing as I age, it is not so much the process of aging itself as the fact that many people I have known much of my life are no longer around. Since Jack and I have a very wide assortment of friends, and since we do not attempt to force our lifestyles onto others, we have some friends who smoke, some who are overweight, some who never exercise. And consequently we have lost a goodly number of friends to heart disease and to cancer.

Cancer is perhaps the most unbearable disease to bear up to, both for the victim and for the victim's friends. Cancer is such a democratic disease: It can strike anyone, and no one is safe from it. You can be the healthiest person in the world and contract cancer. Dr. George Sheehan, the guru of the Running Revolution, a cardiologist, a wonderful writer, and a runner for decades, was struck with cancer. Fortunately, it was diagnosed early and he is still alive and running.

Nothing you can do will guarantee you will not get cancer.

But having said that, let me add that there are things you can do and there are things that you can stop doing that will cut down your chances of getting cancer.

The primary thing is this: If you smoke tobacco, stop. If you chew tobacco, stop. If you use tobacco in any form, stop.

One form of cancer that is of concern to older American men is colon cancer. There is growing evidence that the chances of contracting this form of cancer can be aggravated by diet. As I mentioned before, eating too much fat and cholesterol, especially in the form of red meat, prolongs the passage of food through the intestines. This "stalling" of food in the intestines is detrimental to your health because the longer this fecal matter is stalled in the intestines, the more opportunity it has to do its damage.

Cut down on the amount of fat and cholesterol and increase your intake of fiber-rich foods, drink eight glasses of water a day, eat fresh vegetables and fruits, and exercise regularly, and you'll move those harmful substances through your intestines so they do not have an opportunity to hang around and cause problems.

What types of foods work to prevent cancer? Studies indicate that the orange vegetables are good for this. The beta-carotene in carrots, squash, pumpkins, and other orange fruits and vegetables is excellent. Also, enzymes that fight cancer within the body can be stimulated by brussels sprouts, cauliflower, broccoli, turnips, cabbage, spinach, celery, oranges, grapefruit, lemons, most beans, and various seeds, including sunflower seeds.

At the other end of the spectrum from fresh fruits and vegetables that help deter cancer are the food additives that can lead to cancer: substances put into food for the purpose of giving it a longer shelf life, making it look better, or making it taste better. These additives can be anything from red food dye #4 (which was removed from the market many years ago when it was found to cause cancer in laboratory rats) to sugar and salt. Some additives are taken from nature (cinnamon and cloves, for instance), while others are created to chemically reproduce natural flavors and colors.

Certainly, we are a lot better off these days than we were a century ago. Today, the federal Food and Drug Administration tests additives before they can be used. At the turn of the century, food packagers could put anything they wanted into foods to make them look and taste good—even if by so doing it greatly increased the chances that the food could lead to your demise.

When the government set up its strict additive testing program in 1958, it exempted 670 substances that had been assumed to that point to be safe. Subsequent testing of those 670 substances were made, however, and you'll recall that in 1972 saccharin (a sugar substitute) was removed from the safe list because it was said to contain cancer-causing properties. Saccharin is still used in some diet soft drinks.

One of the greatest potentials for cancer from foods we eat comes from the use of dyes to make foods look more attractive. Many food color dyes have been pulled from use by the Food and Drug Administration because of their cancer-causing properties. Tests are continuing on other dyes. Many of these dyes and colorings are used in junk foods to make them look better than they really are. How can you avoid cancer risks from food dyes? Eat as naturally as you can by using a lot of fresh fruits and vegetables in your diet.

One substance that you'd hope would be safe, but is increasingly questionable, is your drinking water. The presence of certain naturally occurring chemicals in drinking water can become detrimental when they come in contact with chlorine, which is added to public water supplies to purify them. These chemicals could increase the chances of cancer of the kidney, bladder, and the urinary tract. The federal Environmental Protection Agency is currently examining the possibilities of requiring cities to install filtering systems to their water supplies that would remove the potentially harmful chemicals that result from these substances.

In the meantime, home filtering systems can work, but keep in mind the old saying, "You get what you pay for."

"How about bottled water?" you might ask. "It must be safe."

That's not necessarily so. Some bottles of "bottled water" come from the same place as your home water: from the tap.

The safest type of water you can buy is distilled water, which is pure because it is made into steam and all chemicals are removed. Its only drawback is that since everything is removed, it has a rather bland taste. It's the chemicals and minerals in water that give it its taste. Distilled water should not be used exclusively because extended use can leach important minerals from the body.

On the up side of the water and cancer question, many municipal water systems have very good water. Citizens should be aware of the kind of water they are drinking and should take steps to pressure their elected officials to improve the water supply at every turn. For more information about what you should be asking about your public water supply and what you should be demanding, write to the Water Supply Division of the Environmental Protection Agency in Washington, D.C. 20460 and ask for "Manual for Evaluating Public Drinking Water Supplies."

How about alcohol and cancer? Alcohol, although legal, is a drug that can profoundly affect a variety of body organs, including the brain, heart, liver, stomach, and intestines. The highest risk of cancer from alcohol comes to those, logically, who drink the most. What body parts would most likely be affected by alcohol-related cancers? The statistics indicate that cancer of the mouth and throat can be anywhere from double to six times that of nondrinking Americans. Cancer of the larynx is ten times as high, and of the esophagus twenty-five times as high among heavy drinkers as among nondrinkers.

Add cigarette smoking to drinking, and the chance of cancer escalates tremendously because smoking has a way of aggravating any typical problem.

There is also some indication that overconsumption of certain types of alcohol, especially beer and Scotch whiskey, may increase the chances of rectal cancer due to the presence of the nitrate N-nitrosodimethylamine (or NDMA), a potent cancer-causing agent. The nitrate comes from the malt used in the beer and Scotch.

Cancers have also been traced to certain types of teas, especially those that contain sassafras root bark. The types of cancers that can be caused by the tannins in teas are cancers of the esophagus and of the stomach.

Cancer is also caused by obesity. Besides contributing to a variety of other health and medical problems, obesity has been found to contribute to certain cancers in women, among them breast cancer and cancer of the lining of the womb.

What dietary and lifestyle steps, then, can we take to help prevent cancer?

1. Cut down on the amount of dietary fat ingested.
2. Eat fiber (or roughage) every day to keep the bowels regular and clear.
3. Don't smoke.
4. Drink alcohol moderately, if at all.
5. Lose body fat if you are currently overweight.
6. Exercise moderately but regularly.
7. Avoid food additives whenever possible.
8. Eat more fresh fruits and vegetables, especially of the cruciferous family, such as broccoli, brussels sprouts, cauliflower, etc., since these vegetables help prevent certain cancers.
9. Drink juices made from fresh vegetables and fruits.

CONSTIPATION

We've already talked about this problem in the early part of this chapter.

But I would like to stress the fact that I consider constipation harmful to one's health and happiness, and I *do* consider it a disease—but a curable one.

Constipation can literally put your life on hold. If you are constipated you feel miserable and you are giving cancer a chance to get at you.

Jack contends that when a person begins aging, it has nothing to do with calendar age: It has to do with attitude. "You know a person is getting old when the primary topic of the day changes from sex to bowel movements."

Constipation is especially common among older people. And what has the old-age response to constipation been? Get a laxative. Again, this is a *learned* response. We learned this from our mothers. When the bowels are not moving regularly, go to the drugstore and get a laxative. Unfortunately, most laxatives rely for their success on stimulating the colon. Repeated use of a laxative, however, can override the colon's natural reactions. This often leads to a situation where the colon no longer knows how to react on its own.

The best way to increase regularity, and thereby get rid of the chances of developing cancers and other problems associated with constipation, is to:

1. Increase your daily use of high-fiber foods, such as bran.
2. Cut back your intake of red meats, especially red meats high in fat.
3. Increase your daily intake of fresh fruits and vegetables.
4. Do some aerobic exercise at least three times a week, a minimum of twenty minutes per session; this can consist merely of taking a one-mile walk.
5. Drink plenty of water.
6. Instead of using a laxative, try 100 percent pure psyllium husks and/or products containing psyllium. Psyllium products are available in health food stores and some pharmacies.

DEPRESSION

What's this doing here, you ask. Depression is a psychological problem, not one associated with diet. Depression comes from within, not from what you put into your mouth.

Well, that would be the traditional assumption, the assumption we've been taught to believe.

But a person's moods *can* be affected by diet.

In chapter 1 under the topic of sugar, we talked about the tremendous effect that it can have on the human body's energy level, sending it up like a rocket and then dropping like a stone. This drop in energy can often cause depression, because we are weak, we are always tired, we are lazy, and we develop a low opinion of ourselves. Hence, we think we have some sort of deficiency. And we do not realize that it could be due to too much sugar lowering our energy level.

And what happens to many of us when we are depressed?

We look for something to eat.

And then what happens—besides the fact that we add pounds we don't need?

We become even more depressed! A vicious cycle.

What we need in order to avoid depression is habits that make us feel up, alive, self-assured, good about ourselves.

Which person feels better about himself and is less likely to be depressed—the person who has worked up to the ability to walk a mile in fifteen minutes or the person who has added fifteen extra pounds and has trouble getting out of an easy chair without someone else's help? The answer isn't especially difficult, is it?

They say that the rolling stone gathers no moss. I feel that the active body gathers few problems.

How can you possibly be depressed if you are eating well, if you are active, if you are full of energy?

Take control of your life, don't let it take control of you.

1. Eat when you are hungry and not when you aren't. (Remember, you don't want to be Pavlov's dog, you want to be your own person.)
2. Eat what is good for you and your body, and not what you've been "taught" to eat over the years.
3. If you get the urge to eat when you aren't hungry—and who isn't affected by all those food ads on TV?—get up from where you are and take a walk.
4. Eat plenty of fiber and drink plenty of water and you will have a feeling of fullness in your stomach that will help you stay away from food you don't need.
5. Don't eat sugary foods because they will temporarily lift you up and then drop you like a rock, and the drop like a rock can be very, very depressing.
6. When you feel you are becoming depressed, get up and take a walk, or do something else that requires physical activity. You'd be surprised at what a wonderful prescription for health a good walk can be.
7. Don't hang around with other people who are depressing. Spend time with people who are positive and who are enthusiastic about life.
8. Consume plenty of fresh fruits and vegetables.
9. Don't overeat. Take only as large a portion as you feel you can eat. Too much food in your stomach can cause you to feel tired and sluggish, and consequently further depressed.

DIABETES

We've already touched upon diabetes (chapter 1, section 8), a disease that seems to be reaching epidemic proportions in this country, due in large part to our reliance on sugar as a psuedo-food and the tendency of the average American to be overfat. It never hurts to review a subject, so let's take a brief look at the two types of diabetes and then we'll examine how diet affects the disease.

When you eat, insulin is delivered to the bloodstream to connect up with the sugar released from the food you have just digested. The insulin moves glucose to the cells to be used as energy.

If you do not produce adequate insulin or if your body cannot make use of insulin, the transfer of glucose from your bloodstream to your cells does not happen, and the sugar remains in your bloodstream and your body runs down from lack of fuel.

There are two types of diabetes:

Type I involves people who produce little or no insulin in their bodies. This type of diabetes makes up about 10 percent of the people who have diabetes, and it generally sets in during childhood.

Type II diabetes constitutes 90 percent of those with the disease. When there are not enough insulin receptors available, glucose cannot get to the cells and it builds up in the bloodstream. Unlike Type I diabetes, which comes on typically during childhood, Type II develops gradually, and often has its onset in adulthood.

Let's look at the possible causes of Type II diabetes:

1. Age, especially over forty.
2. Overweight (overfat).
3. Poor eating habits.
4. Had diabetes during pregnancy.
5. Family history of diabetes.

Now let's look at some of the symptoms of Type II diabetes, keeping in mind that some people may have these symptoms to a lesser extent than others, and some may not have them at all yet still have the disease. It should also be noted that because a person has one or two of these symptoms, it is not an indication of diabetes. Always consult your doctor when in doubt.

1. Increased hunger.
2. Increased thirst.
3. Increased urination.
4. Blurred eyesight.
5. Chronic fatigue.
6. Numbness or tingling in hands or feet.
7. Frequent infections.
8. Slow healing of cuts or sores.
9. Impotence and other sexual problems.

What are the methods of treating Type II diabetes? There are five primary tools:

1. Meal planning—proper meals at the right time, attention to calories, and losing body fat.

2. Physical activity—daily exercise promotes your body's ability to use its own insulin, and assists in fat loss.

3. Medication—usually involves taking an oral hypoglycemic agent to help you more effectively use insulin.

4. Self-monitoring—this involves a person closely monitoring blood glucose levels.

5. Education—by learning exactly what is happening within your body, or what is *not* happening, a diabetic is more likely to be able to effect a "cure."

Now let's take a look at what dietary rules are necessary to control Type II diabetes:

Eat well-balanced meals. A variety of good foods every day gives your body the nutrition it needs to function properly, while also regulating your body fat.

Eat meals and snacks as scheduled. As opposed to the person who must fight the urge to eat because it is time to eat (see chapter 1, section 5), the Type II diabetic *must* eat smaller meals but more frequently in order to better use the body's insulin. This scheduled dietary manipulation is necessary in order to maintain a glucose-insulin level. It is also important for losing weight, since eating more often but in smaller amounts tends to make the diabetic feel fuller during the day, making it less likely that he or she will snack.

Eat more fiber. Fiber assists in lowering blood glucose levels.

Eat less sugar. Sugar has no food value, lots of calories, and no vitamins or minerals. And it plays havoc with your glucose levels, and consequently with your insulin production.

Eat less animal fat. Too much animal fat leads to heart problems, too much body fat, and high blood pressure—all of which further complicate your diabetes problems.

Eat less salt. Salt causes water retention, which leads to high blood pressure.

HEART DISEASE

This topic alone could be the subject for a whole separate book—and has often been just that. Plain and simply, heart disease is the number one killer of adult Americans.

There are ten factors that contribute to heart disease; some we have control over, others we do not.

The factors over which we have no control are these:

Heredity
Sex
Age

Most of the factors that contribute to heart disease are factors over which we do have varying degrees of control. These are the factors:

High blood cholesterol
High blood pressure
Cigarette smoking
Diabetes
Obesity
Vascular disease
Stress

Many of these factors over which we have some control are linked. For instance, if a person is obese and inactive, his or her chances of having diabetes are increased, as are the chances of suffering from high blood pressure and high blood cholesterol. Unfortunately, with heart disease, each time that you combine several of these factors in one person, the chances of developing heart disease increases many-fold.

High blood cholesterol, high blood pressure, and cigarette smoking are the three most significant risk factors for heart disease. Cigarette smoking is a voluntary vice, which is controllable. High blood pressure is often a symptom of various other problems, frequently involving obesity, inactivity, and high cholesterol.

Cholesterol has gotten a lot of attention over the last few years because increasingly studies of heart disease indicate that blood serum cholesterol numbers are valid indicators of a person's likelihood of developing serious heart disease.

Most heart disease does not really involve the heart directly. It is caused by the clogging of blood vessels going to and from the heart. Think of your kitchen sink drain as an artery. If it is filled with saturated fats, it becomes clogged. The arteries also become clogged with plaque generated by too much cholesterol in the foods you eat and too much inactivity. When the blood vessels clog, the blood supply to the heart is restricted and the arteries literally starve and choke the heart for lack of oxygen, sometimes resulting in death.

Cholesterol levels *can* be changed by diet and exercise. They are not the only factors influencing a person's blood cholesterol level, but they are among the most easily changed.

The principal factors involved in cholesterol are:

Diet
Weight
Physical activity/exercise
Genetic factors
Sex/age
Stress

By learning how these factors interact, you will have a better understanding of cholesterol and how it affects you and your chances of developing heart disease.

Diet. Cholesterol levels are raised by eating saturated fats. Period. Also, cholesterol in your diet increases cholesterol in your blood. The good news is that you can control your diet to lower your cholesterol. Food manufacturers have been responding to the increasing knowledge of how cholesterol and saturated fats in the diet work to increase your serum cholesterol, and they've been making more and more foods available with lower or no saturated fats and lower or no cholesterol.

Weight. A person who is overfat often has high cholesterol because of a poor diet and inactivity. Lower the body fat and the cholesterol level is lowered.

Physical activity/exercise. Regular aerobic exercise controls body fat, lowers blood pressure, and increases HDL (high density lipoprotein, the "good" cholesterol that scrubs away the LDL, low density lipoprotein, or "bad" cholesterol).

Genetic factors. A person's cholesterol level is determined to a large extent by heredity factors. Studies show that roughly 75 percent of a person's cholesterol level is determined by genetic factors. It is the remaining 25 percent that a person can manipulate downward by diet and exercise and by other lifestyle changes.

Sex/age. Before they reach the age of sixty, one out of every five men and one out of every seventeen women in this country will have developed some symptoms of heart disease. Men are at much higher risk for heart disease than women, and the older a person becomes, the higher the risk. In women, serum cholesterol levels rise significantly after menopause until the numbers sometimes go beyond those of men.

Stress. People increase their serum cholesterol levels during periods of high stress. However, it is not known precisely why.

Fortunately, making lifestyle changes as far as diet and exercise are concerned can have a *significant* effect upon cholesterol levels, and consequently on lowering heart disease.

Since the 1970s, there have been some heart disease clinics that have actually had marathon-training programs for people who have suffered heart attacks. The fact that these people changed from the typical American lifestyle to the lifestyle of a marathoner accounts for their very high success rate in pushing back or preventing that second (and often fatal) heart attack that frequently follows a first heart attack.

I do not intend to push anyone to take up a marathon lifestyle, but making some basic dietary changes and adding exercise to your life can make a world of difference, while adding years to your life and quality to those years.

HIGH BLOOD PRESSURE

Hypertension, or high blood pressure, is epidemic among adult Americans. High blood pressure can cause heart disease, kidney disease, and stroke. As a rule, one of the most common causes of high blood pressure is obesity. And when one is overweight or overfat, the following complications can occur.

Your heart has to work overtime to force blood throughout your body when the passageways are restricted; varicose veins are more common; the chances of gout increase; you have less energy and become more tired; the bones and joints undergo more weight loads with each movement; the lungs are restricted so that breathing becomes more difficult; and diabetes is more likely to develop.

And ironically, often the overweight person is undernourished, in spite of the number of calories taken in each day, because the calories taken in are often hollow calories that are of no nutritional value whatsoever.

What can a person do who is overweight and suffering from high blood pressure? This may sound like a broken record, but here goes:

1. Cut down on the ingestion of salt.
2. Consume fiber on a regular basis.
3. Cut out sweets.
4. Stop eating processed foods, such as lunch meat and frozen dinners.
5. Get up and move around on a regular basis. Strive to walk one mile a day for starters.

Most high blood pressure and obesity are avoidable. And when you begin doing the five things outlined above on a daily basis, you'll be surprised at what a lift you'll get out of life as you begin to feel better and look better, and as the person trapped inside you is allowed to come out and be seen.

INSOMNIA

Scientists who study sleep still are not certain why people need it. Of course, we can tell scientists why *we* need sleep: to allow ourselves to become rested and restored. Yet insomnia—or lack of restful, restorative sleep—is so common and so debilitating to so many people that I consider it a disease.

Are you one of those many people who can't remember the last time they've had a good night's sleep and feel it is just something that comes with aging?

When I talk with people about their sleep patterns, I find that some simple diet and lifestyle changes would do wonders to restore the bliss of a good night's sleep.

Let's deal with lack of sleep as though it were a disease just like any of the other diseases on this list. Let's examine a string of factors that could be contributing to insomnia.

Coffee, tea, or chocolate. Do you drink coffee or tea or hot chocolate or eat chocolates in the evening? Coffee, most teas, hot chocolate, and chocolates contain caffeine. Caffeine is a stimulant and will wire you, which will in turn keep you awake when you are trying to go to sleep. Try cutting out coffee, tea, hot chocolate, and chocolates after 5 P.M.

Alcohol. Consuming one ounce of alcohol in the evening may have a soothing effect, since alcohol is a depressant. But too much alcohol can interfere with your REM (rapid eye movement) or dream sleep, and although you will fall asleep quickly after overimbibing, you may wake up a few hours later and be unable to get back to sleep. Cut back on your alcohol to no more than one ounce, which translates into one 12-ounce can of beer, one glass of wine, or one shot of hard liquor, or better yet, cut out drinking entirely.

Cigarettes. Don't smoke cigarettes, period. But if you do, smoking cigarettes after dinner can also hinder your sleep because nicotine can have a stimulating effect, which makes it difficult to become relaxed.

Eating too late. Some people can sleep like a baby after eating late, but it can sometimes inhibit your sleep. The interference can come not only from *what* and how much you eat, but from your stomach's ability to process the food. If you have insomnia, eat your evening meal early, and forget the snacks before bedtime.

Stress. Stress, whether it's stress at the office, stress at home, or personal anxieties, can prevent a good night's sleep. The best way I know of to relieve stress is not a pill—it is exercise. After your evening meal, instead of sitting around stewing about the things in your life that are bothering you, take a walk for a half-hour, or do some exercises from my books *Dynastride!* or *The Fitness After 50 Workout*. The exercise relieves physical stress, helps digestion, relieves psychological stress, and a brisk walk or some exercise routine often helps you solve life's problems by simplifying things. And remember the adage that a good idea never comes while you're sitting down. Exercising right before bedtime can be relaxing for some and put them to sleep, but for others, exercise gets the blood pumping and the oxygen in the body has a reviving effect. So if you have a sleeping problem, exercise a few hours before bedtime. That will allow the good effects of exercise to be absorbed by the body, and will promote restful sleep.

OBESITY

It seems as if we've discussed this subject over and over in this chapter because of its contributions to other diseases such as diabetes and heart disease.

Obesity is considered by many experts to be a disease, and I agree. Obesity contributes to so many other problems that it should be ranked among the most pervasive and influential diseases in our country today. Unfortunately, in spite of the fact that a record number of Americans are taking up a fitness lifestyle, record numbers of Americans are also overfat. Despite the fact that we have accumulated so much knowledge relative to diet and nutrition, Americans are still eating more of what they shouldn't.

My Dad was an example of a person who was overfat. I can still hear him say, "I need some food that will stick to my ribs." And he often thought I needed more "meat on my bones."

Today we know that carrying a lot of weight around does not indicate good health unless that weight is composed of good solid muscle. Unfortunately, when people used to use the expression "meat on the bones," they weren't really talking about meat (which is muscle), they were talking about fat.

Our idea that a pudgy infant is a healthy infant has been proven incorrect. Frequently, the pudgy infant becomes the obese adult.

Some statistics have been gathered to prove that obese children come from obese parents, but obese children more frequently come from parents who have unwise eating habits and little or no exercise habits.

A person who has reached sixty years of age in this country has often done so while adding a mere pound of excess fat per year. By age sixty, that's sixty pounds of unnecessary fat that is interfering with all sorts of critical bodily functions, from causing high blood pressure and heart disease, to putting a strain on the lower back and on the weight-bearing joints in the ankles and legs.

This is the gift you can give to yourself by shedding that excess weight: blood pressure drops, arteries slow their clogging, the chances of diabetes drops significantly, joints and muscles ache less from carrying around what amounts to a knapsack filled with sixty pounds of stones. Remember that "less is more": The less excess weight you carry around, the more you are doing for yourself and the more you'll get out of life.

Here are the basic essentials necessary for losing excess body fat:

1. Break out of bad nutritional habits.
2. Develop a set of good nutritional habits.
3. Exercise regularly.
4. Eat more good food.
5. Try juicing fresh fruits and vegetables as a healthy substitute for the high and hollow calories in soft drinks.

Ironically, the exercising person can—and does—consume more calories per day than the overfat person, yet is often 20 percent lighter than that person.

Give yourself the gift of life by taking away the fat that is dragging you down. I'd like to suggest two of my previous exercise books: *Dynastride!* and *The Fitness After 50 Workout.* The first presents an easy-to-follow walking program, while the second presents programs aimed at slimming down and shaping up specific body parts.

Disease in America is frustrating to me because so many of the diseases that bedevil and often kill Americans are diseases of choice.

By that I mean that we make choices in our lives that make us vulnerable to certain diseases. For instance, if we choose to smoke cigarettes we subject ourselves to lung disease and heart disease. If we allow ourselves to become overweight, we are prone to high blood pressure, heart disease, diabetes, etc.

As I look at this great country of ours, I am increasingly disappointed and disillusioned at how many people want to lay the blame for their own mistakes on other things and other people.

Often we do not want to accept responsibility for our actions. We tend to want to blame something or someone else for our problems. I've heard these lines time and again:

"But I can't help it."

"I'm too busy."

"I'm too tired."

"I'm too old."

"I have no will power."

"The devil made me do it."

At some point, if we really care about ourselves, we must take responsibility and break old habits and begin thinking in new ways.

Today can be the day you look in the mirror and say, "Enough, already! I'm my own person. I'm taking back control of my life. I'm going to eat right, exercise, and enjoy a more active lifestyle. I'm going to increase the quantity *and* the quality of my life by eating good foods, avoiding bad foods, and distancing myself as much as possible from the most likely American diseases that Elaine outlined. I'm in control here! I'm declaring today my own Independence Day! My old way of life is out the window!"

Vitamin and Mineral Supplements: Yes or No?

We've come a long way since I was a child. I don't even remember seeing a vitamin pill until I was grown. The only thing I remember about vitamins is that when he was a young man, my father suffered from rickets and scurvy. So my mother made sure we had fresh orange juice every day. She also insisted we take cod liver oil. But that's about all I remember about vitamins and minerals until I was pregnant with my first child, Danny. The doctor recommended certain vitamins.

He did this because my diet was so poor and deficient in essential vitamins and minerals that there were not enough of either to sustain both the child I was carrying and myself. Consequently, my body elected to nourish my unborn Danny, and I came up short. This condition caused a lack of vitamins and minerals, especially calcium. That deficiency resulted in a dozen decaying teeth. The decaying teeth caused every joint in my body to act as though they were suffering from arthritis. I couldn't even lift my hands over my head and couldn't even dress myself, the pain was so overwhelming.

The doctor recommended vitamin supplements and that I go to see my dentist. After the dentist filled my teeth, my pains left me. I couldn't believe the far-reaching effects a lack of sufficient vitamins and minerals could have on the human body.

We know, for instance, that *a lack of certain vitamins* can open the door to disease. Rickets is caused by a lack of vitamin D, while scurvy is caused by a lack of vitamin C in the diet.

Some people feel that we get all the vitamins and minerals we need from a balanced diet. I would agree with that. Unfortunately, many Americans do not eat a balanced diet. According to The Council for Responsible Nutrition, the following is a list of the groups most at risk from a lack of sufficient vitamins and minerals.

Dieters. Each year in America, some fifty million people are on some sort of diet. These diets are often fad diets or nutritionally unsafe diets. Consequently, these people may not receive their daily vitamin and mineral requirements.

Alcoholics. There are ten million problem drinkers in the country, and they usually have very inadequate diets, which further speeds the deterioriating effects of their drinking problems. It takes a tremendous amount of B vitamins to help counter the heavy drinking. These people almost never get the daily requirements of vitamins and minerals, and their bodies suffer as a consequence.

The elderly. Some twenty-five million elderly Americans do not enjoy a balanced diet, the result of a variety of reasons.

1. Poor teeth and therefore an inability to eat certain foods.
2. Obstructed digestion due to irregularity or stomach problems.
3. Poverty (and an inability to afford sufficient amounts of good food).
4. Medications that kill the appetite and therefore prevent them getting sufficient nourishment.
5. Diminished interest in eating (as one ages, the taste buds dull) and sometimes even forgetfulness about eating regularly.

Many of these time-honored Americans are not getting sufficient vitamins and minerals from their diet—just at a time when they may need them most.

Women. There are millions of older women in this country who are suffering from malnutrition due to maintaining daily diets in the range of 1,400 to 1,600 calories. Often, these 1,600 calories are lacking in the good nutrition necessary to maintain good health. Their minimum daily requirement of vitamins and minerals is not coming from the food they eat.

From my own observation, I would also add that many American businessmen and businesswomen of all ages often eat fatty business lunches, eat at their desks, eat on the run, or forget to eat at all. Their diets are often deficient in vitamins and minerals.

Also, people who are either physically active or who have recently gone through an illness are also frequently down on their needed vitamins and minerals, and probably need some sort of supplementation.

There have been surveys conducted to figure out just how many Americans regularly take vitamins and mineral supplements. The numbers are rather impressive, and the findings indicate that over half of the vitamin users in this country fall into two age groups: young people under eighteen and mature Americans fifty-nine years of age and above.

A Gallup Poll survey indicated that 37 percent of the adult population of the United States takes vitamin supplements. Of that 37 percent, 68 percent of them take multivitamins, 32 percent take vitamin C, 27 percent take B vitamins, 20 percent take vitamin E, and 19 percent take minerals.

The same survey indicated that the Americans who take vitamin supplements are of a higher demographic group than those who do not. John L. Stanton, Ph.D., analyzed the Gallup report in an issue of *Vitamin Issues* and has this to say about vitamin supplement users:

"Vitamin supplement usage is greater among women than men (especially full-time working women); among college graduates than high school graduates or non-graduates; and among professional, clerical, and sales people than manual laborers or those not in the work force at all. There is greater usage in the $10,000 + income groups and in households without children living at home. Finally, vitamin supplement usage is more common in the West than in any other area of the country."

The vitamin and mineral supplement business has grown at an incredible rate, indicating that many Americans have chosen to supplement the vitamins and minerals provided to them in their diets. The Stanford Research Institute reported that sales of vitamin and mineral supplements were $500 million in 1972, $1.2 billion in 1980, and $3.5 billion in 1988.

Most people who take multivitamin supplements report that they do so either to supplement their diet or because they feel it is the healthy thing to do and that it makes them feel better.

In a 1984 report on a survey of dietitians in Washington State, nearly 60 percent of the respondents reported that they used some form of dietary supplementation.

In spite of the support of using vitamin and mineral supplements, there are still some very loud critics of the practice. In their book *Vitamins and "Health" Foods: The Great American Hustle*, Drs. Victor Herbert and Stephen Barrett stated their case this way:

"Suggestions to take vitamins seem to be everywhere. Advertisements on radio and television and in magazines and newspapers warn against deficiencies. Self-appointed 'experts,' echoed by a chorus of believers, praise the 'miracles' of nutrition. Colorful bottles line the shelves—not only in health food stores but also in pharmacies, supermarkets, and department stores. Doctors even prescribe vitamins as placebos."

Unfortunately, in some of what they say, I would tend to agree with Drs. Herbert and Barrett.

Some vitamin and mineral supplement manufacturers *do* go overboard in their advertising and their claims and, I think, do more harm than good in their efforts to grab a segment of the increasing supplement market.

Fortunately, most of the supplements from major producers are very much aboveboard, and considering the way Americans eat—or don't eat—quite a few experts have come around to the view that the regular use of supplements will not harm you, and will in many instances help you. I have been using vitamin supplements since 1953 and feel that they are essential in my life. I have found that as I age, vitamin supplements are even more critical to maintaining my active lifestyle.

Dr. Willard A. Krehl, in an issue of *Vitamin Issues,* has this to say about supplements in an article he titles "Vitamin Supplementation—A Practical View":

"Thus it comes as no surprise to me that national surveys reflect the nutritional imbalances and micronutrient shortages they do. It's not that the food supply is deficient; the 'deficiency' lies in people's ability or motivation to use food properly.

"I strongly favor multivitamin supplementation and recommend it to my patients because I believe it is a simple, economical, and highly practical way to insure they receive 100 percent of the RDA for essential micronutrients, and because I believe these intakes are important to health and well being."

Dr. Krehl, using various surveys of the eating habits of Americans, estimates conservatively that some 23 million Americans are regularly getting less than 70 percent of the RDA. Vitamin and mineral supplements can serve to effectively cut down that number of what I feel are undernourished Americans.

Some critics of vitamin and mineral supplements warn about the toxic effects of taking too many vitamin and mineral supplements. It is true that there are certain vitamins and minerals you don't want to overdo, such as vitamin A. But to overdo it, you would have to take tremendous amounts. For instance, the recommended daily adult intake of vitamin A is 5,000 IU (International Unit), while a MTD (minimum toxic dose) would be between 25,000 and 50,000 IU. For vitamin D, the recommended adult intake is 400 IU, while the MTD is 50,000 IU.

There are some people who feel that if one is good, ten must be ten times as good, and some of these people *do* occasionally overdo it with vitamins. But to overdo it, as you can see, you've really got to go out of your way. Just remember not to overdo vitamin A. Also remember the famous LaLanneism: "If one apple a day is good for you, you wouldn't eat a hundred, would you?"

A person taking a multivitamin on a daily basis is not going to run into these problems.

Jane Brody, the very popular and very knowledgeable science and medical writer for *The New York Times,* has this to say about vitamin-mineral supplement needs in her book *Jane Brody's Nutrition Book* (revised edition), published in 1987:

"Persons most likely to need a vitamin-mineral supplement are those consuming fewer than 1,500 calories a day; those who, for health reasons, must eliminate a major category of food from their diets (for example, all dairy products or fresh fruit and vegetables); or those taking medications that interfere with the body's ability to absorb or use certain vitamins or minerals. Chronic use of laxatives, antibiotics, antacids, diuretics, oral diabetes drugs, some anti-inflammatory drugs, and certain cancer drugs, among others, can result in a depletion of essential vitamins and minerals."

Susan Male Smith, M.A., R.D., feels that "what the public wants is *advice* on supplementation, not lectures." Her approach is very even-handed, and in her article "A New Approach to Vitamin Supplementation" in the April 1984 issue of *Environmental Nutrition Newsletter,* Ms. Smith gives some very good guidelines for choosing a vitamin supplement:

> The following guidelines can help consumers choose a safe and effective preparation for their money:
>
> 1. Choose a balanced multi-vitamin, rather than one or two specific nutrients, unless it has been medically prescribed. (Excessive levels of one nutrient can disrupt the body's balance and actually alter nutrient requirements. In addition, one is rarely deficient or suboptimal in one nutrient; usually several are involved.)
> 2. Choose a preparation that provides at least 100 percent of the RDA (Recommended Daily Allowances) for *recognized* nutrients, in approximately equal proportions.
> 3. Avoid preparations containing unrecognized nutrients, or nutrients in minute amounts (this only increases the cost, but is of no real value).
> 4. Do research on preparations that claim to be 'natural,' 'organic,' 'therapeutic,' 'high-potency,' or for 'stress' (the extra cost is not worth any purported benefit; many unreputable firms use these claims, and thus may signal less effective preparations).
> 5. Beware of 'natural' versus 'synthetic' claims; they are sometimes meaning-

less. Certain synthetic vitamin preparations are occasionally *more* effective than their natural counterparts.

6. Choose a preparation with an expiration date on it. Certain nutrients interact with others (e.g., thiamin actually hastens the decomposition of both folate and vitamin B-12). As a result, vitamin preparations lose potency with time and hot, humid environments, such as bathrooms, accelerate this process.

It is important to have a working knowledge of just how much of each essential vitamin and mineral a person should take each day in order to sustain good health and to ward off diseases associated with vitamin and mineral deficiencies. The chart below is an adpation of the 1989 revision of the Recommended Dietary Allowances, which is prepared by the Food and Nutrition Board of the National Academy of Sciences. Do not let the chart overwhelm you. Merely find your sex and age range and then follow it to the specific vitamin or mineral. The amounts are given in one of the following units of measure: g = gram, mg = milligram, and µg = microgram. On a package of vitamin and mineral supplements, the units of measurement will be similar or identical.

	Male			Female		
	19-24	25-50	51+	19-24	25-50	51+
Protein (g)	58	63	63	46	50	50
Vit.A (µg)	1000	1000	1000	800	800	800
Vit.D (µg)	10	5	5	10	5	5
Vit.E (mg)	10	10	10	8	8	8
Vit.K (µg)	70	80	80	60	65	65
Vit.C (mg)	60	60	60	60	60	60
Thiamin (mg)	1.5	1.5	1.2	1.1	1.1	1.0
Riboflavin (mg)	1.7	1.7	1.4	1.3	1.3	1.2
Niacin (mg)	19	19	15	15	15	13
Vit.B6 (mg)	2.0	2.0	2.0	1.6	1.6	1.6
Folate (µg)	200	200	200	180	180	180
Vit.B12 (µg)	2.0	2.0	2.0	2.0	2.0	2.0
Calcium (mg)	1200	800	800	1200	800	800
Phosphorus (mg)	1200	800	800	1200	800	800
Magnesium (mg)	350	350	350	280	280	280
Iron (mg)	10	10	10	15	15	10
Zinc (mg)	15	15	15	12	12	12
Iodine (µg)	150	150	150	150	150	150
Selenium (µg)	70	70	70	55	55	55

The Special Nutritional and Exercise Needs of the 50-Plus American

It is no big news to the person over fifty years of age that as the human body ages, it goes through certain distinct periods where it makes rather dramatic changes.

The infant seems to do little more than sleep and eat, the result of the tremendous metabolism at work to power the rapid growth spurts that the little body experiences. The teenage years are marked by similar high metabolic levels and growth spurts that are sometimes startling.

During the twenties and thirties the metabolic furnaces cut back considerably because most of the growth is finished; the metabolism is now concerned with repairing and maintaining the body and with fueling its movements. (A physically active body stokes the fires in the body's metabolism, which is how exercisers burn off unwanted calories.)

When you reach the forties your metabolism seems to further slow down and you can see changes in certain body functions: eyesight often starts to deteriorate, it is easier to put on body fat (and more difficult to get rid of it), occasional constipation may occur, minor or selective hearing loss may develop, etc.

Beyond fifty years of age, the metabolism begins to dampen its fires, the proportion of muscle to fat in the body changes gradually in favor of the fat, bone density begins to leach away, the teeth and gums can more easily develop problems, eyesight is more seriously affected, muscles stiffen and overall flexibility diminishes, and digestive problems often occur.

These are the inevitable processes of aging that happen within the human body pretty much the same way it happens within a car or a house: Parts wear down, rafters warp, steps creak.

Although the aging process is inevitable, we do have some control over the speed with which it happens to each of us.

A deserted house deteriorates faster than one that is lived in and maintained. A car that sits in the weeds out behind the garage ages faster than one that is driven and that is stored inside the garage.

That is why at seventy years of age, Jack LaLanne could tow seventy boats filled with seventy people one and a half miles from the Queen's Way Bridge in Long Beach Harbor to the Queen Mary while handcuffed and shackled—this at the same point in time that other seventy-year-olds were bedridden. As Jack always says, "I'd rather wear out than rust out."

There must be some logical explanation for the huge gulf between Jack towing seventy boats and another seventy-year-old lying helplessly in a hospital or nursing home bed.

The saying that "You are what you eat" comes to mind here, and many Americans beyond fifty years of age could make a tremendous change in their lives if they would feed themselves a balanced meal.

It seems that there is a process that afflicts a person beyond fifty years of age, but especially beyond sixty. Life begins to dictate to us, instead of allowing us to dictate to it.

People we have known all our lives die and are no longer available to us, retirement looms, we become more susceptible to certain illnesses, our movements tend to be somewhat restricted by our physical limitations (we are not likely to take up sky diving at age sixty the way we might have at age twenty-five, for instance), we tend to be generally more cautious on one hand and more foolish on the other.

In other words, we allow life to push us around, to herd us into pens that match our age. Who's in charge here?

Of course, *we don't have to allow that process to occur.* But many people do. In essence, they seem to surrender to what they see as the inevitable: brittle bones, quiet little meals alone, reduced horizons, periodic or ongoing depression, bouts of nostalgia—of how it used to be, but no longer is.

As I write this, there are 30 million Americans sixty-five years of age or older. Many of these 30 million Americans are living highly restricted lives, not because they have to, but because they feel it is expected of them because they are old.

They see themselves as fragile and ineffective and, because they see themselves that way, they are that way. It is the self-fulfilling prophecy at its worst.

On the other hand, there are many older people who are extremely active. I enjoy each month reading a section in the back of *Runner's World* magazine called "The Human Race," in which the magazine's editors highlight very special athletes, many of whom are fifty and above. I have before me the October 1990 issue. Meet three 50-plus Americans who somehow forgot to let their age tell them that they should sit back and wait for the inevitable:

Jim Hodge is fifty years old. He ran track back in his high school days at Haverford High School in Pennsylvania, but when he left high school, he left track behind—until he turned forty. At forty he took up track again, and now runs for the Philadelphia Masters Club, where he is vice-president. "The competitiveness at this age is just amazing," he said. And, get this: He can still run a quarter-mile in sixty seconds!

Norman Frank is fifty-nine years old, and over the past twenty-three years has run more than 400 marathons. In 1983 alone, he ran thirty-five marathons and eleven races longer than the marathon. He does this in spite of having an arthritic left hip. Somebody forgot to tell Norman that he can't do this kind of thing, that he's too old.

Margaret Lee is seventy years old. A native Hawaiian, Margaret didn't begin running until 1975. She ran her first marathon in 1977; it took her more than six hours, but the next year she ran the same marathon and knocked an hour off it. And in 1983, she had her time down to 4:11. At the 1990 Los Angeles International Marathon, Margaret set a national age group record for the 70 to 74 age group with a 4:31.

Or how about the competitors in the Senior Olympics?

Dr. John Williams was a spry seventy-eight when he competed in the second U.S. National Senior Olympics in 1988. He had won a bronze medal in the breaststroke in the 1987 Games. Dr. Williams is a retired public health professor from Appalachian State University in Boone, North Carolina. "If you contrast swimming with other healthful activities like running or jogging or even walking, swimming is the winner every time because of buoyancy," he contends. "There is no pressure on the joints and tendons. And an aerobic workout is good for your heart, lungs, and cardiovascular system."

Is aging inevitable? Yes. But do we have something to say about how quickly "inevitable" comes along? Ask Jim Hodge, Norman Frank, Margaret Lee, and John Williams.

By eating well and by getting out there and moving around under our own power, we *can* slow the inevitable aging. And no, you don't have to run seventy miles a week and compete with Margaret Lee in order to enjoy a fulfilling life after fifty.

This chapter concerns eating well and exercising to get the full measure of pleasure out of your years beyond fifty. Let's get out the knives and forks and the walking shoes and get into it!

MALNUTRITION: THE DISEASE OF THE ELDERLY

Would it shock you to know that nearly 40 percent of the elderly in America are suffering from malnutrition—even though they eat three meals a day?

And I am not referring to malnutrition merely among the poor. The middle class and the affluent older person can be just as malnourished as the poorest person.

How can this be?

How can someone who is eating three meals a day be malnourished?

In a society where packaged food is so readily available, it can happen very easily.

When does this happen?

Usually when life causes a person over fifty to make compromises.

If a woman of sixty-two has been making nutritious meals for herself and her husband all their married life, and the husband suddenly dies, the structure of her life is very much altered.

Besides going through a period of depression and disorientation to her new situation, she may just plain forget to eat. She's not likely to go to the trouble to cook for herself; her period of grief and depression from losing her life's mate will imprint new eating habits on her lifestyle.

With the motivation for creating meals gone from her life, she will likely "make do" with conveniently packaged and undernourishing meals. I'm sympathetic to this, because when Jack is out of town, I often find my interest in cooking a nutritious meal is just not there. For the person alone, this dilemma can take on tragic proportions.

Meals will now come out of cans or they'll be TV dinners. Instead of eating fresh fruits and vegetables and well-prepared chicken and meats, those alone will be inclined to eat highly processed food that is low in nutrients, high in salt and sugar, low in fibers and starches, and high in fat and cholesterol.

It is unfortunate that many people in this situation are told that this deterioration is part and parcel of aging when, in fact, it is frequently a matter of improper diet. A lack of certain vitamins and minerals found in a balanced diet can lead to anemia, and can also contribute to senility, which, left to go too long, can effectively put an end to one's life as an independent person, and ultimately to institutionalization. These people invariably begin to feel fragile and weak, and as a result, they cut way back on any type of physical activity, one of the very things that could pull them back onto the healthy, productive path.

PHYSICAL CHANGES CAUSED BY AGING, AND THEIR DIETARY SOLUTIONS

If you don't take care of yourself, you will find that when your body passes the age of fifty it has changed to a different configuration from what it was ten or twenty years before, and it could very well get away from you.

As we age:

1. Our metabolism slows; we need to eat fewer total calories per day, both because we are usually less active, and because our body has been gradually changing its proportion of muscle to fat. Fat requires fewer calories to maintain, since the fat is essentially available calorie reserves. Caloric needs are down, so if you have been in the habit of eating 2,500 calories per day, you are going to store the excess calories as fat. There is therefore a tendency to more easily put on weight as we age, with a corresponding difficulty in getting it off.

2. We can become victims of depression if we allow ourselves to become too passive. A typical reaction to depression among some people is to attempt to eat away the doldrums—usually with an assault of chocolates or a barrage of junk food . . . or a binge of alcohol.

3. If we don't take care of ourselves, our teeth can go bad on us, and eating an apple a day (remember the adage of "An apple a day . . ."?) becomes more difficult—as does eating any type of roughage. Consequently, we do not get our daily ration of fiber, and when we don't, we tend to become irregular.

   Instead of laxatives, keep plenty of roughage in your diet: fresh fruit, bran (especially in the form of hot cereals at breakfast), fresh salads with plenty of fresh vegetables.

   By filling your diet with fresh fruits and vegetables, as you age you will also supply your body with many of the vitamins it needs.

4. I might mention here that as we age, our tolerance for caffeine diminishes. If you are having trouble sleeping, this may be the problem. Avoid drinking caffeinated coffee between lunch and bedtime. The same goes for tea and chocolate. Chocolate also contains caffeine, and some teas have more caffeine than coffee. Be sure

to read the labels on any soft drinks you consume; many soft drinks contain caffeine. You may associate caffeine with the cola drinks, but did you know that some of the clear soft drinks contain more caffeine than the average cola?

5. We also have a tendency to process proteins incompletely, so keep up your ingestion of protein. Remember, however, that you can get protein from a lot of different sources other than meat, which has a high fat content.

6. Our body's ability to pull vitamins and minerals from the food we eat is somewhat hindered, so it is important to provide an adequate supply of vitamins and minerals. That is why I feel confident in recommending that the average person over fifty consider taking a multivitamin plus iron every day.

   Do not take megadoses of vitamins except under the direction of your physician. Certain vitamins, such as vitamin A, taken in megadoses can have harmful effects.

7. Calcium in your diet is important in order to keep your bones dense and healthy.

   There are other sources of calcium besides milk, and the one that is my favorite is broccoli. Broccoli contains large amounts of calcium and can be used in a variety of ways: in fresh salads, soups, stews, and as a side dish. If it is cooked, it should be cooked lightly so that it retains its crispness and its dark green color.

   Your calcium intake will help prevent osteoporosis, or bone loss. It will also help prevent periodontal diseases, which are diseases where the bones that support the teeth begin to deteriorate. Be sure to get a sufficient amount of calcium in your diet, be sure to brush and floss your teeth regularly, and you can help prevent periodontal disease, while also retarding osteoporosis.

8. Osteoporosis is more prevalent. It is a disease in which bone density deteriorates. It is as though there were termites in your bones, eating away at the solid structure of the bone, filling it with microscopic holes, until the bones can no longer support your weight. They begin to fracture easily, and they tend to shrink in upon themselves, which accounts for some elderly people seeming to shrink as they age. It is also a contributing factor to the feeling of being fragile and breakable.

   Studies conducted over the past decade have found that regular aerobic exercise increases bone density, but exercise is something we'll get into with the next section of this chapter.

9. Fat and cholesterol become more of a concern. If you could cut your fat down to 5 percent of your diet or less, you'd be so much better off. The same is true of cholesterol. Some people are of the opinion that once you are beyond a certain age—let's say sixty—that diet modifications have very little effect. That just is *not* true. The research has shown that people above sixty who modify their cholesterol intake downward have enjoyed lowered blood cholesterol, and it is believed that the built-up plaque clogging the insides of their arteries actually begins to recede. So don't ever swallow that old saying that "You can't teach an old dog new tricks." Old dogs are often wise dogs, and a wise dog knows that a new trick may be just what he needs to turn his life around and to liven up his days.

As I write this, there is a movement to regulate the claims of diet pill manufacturers and purveyors. An incredible number of Americans, primarily women, have become addicted to diet pills. Some of the diet pills require prescriptions, others can be purchased over-the-counter or by mail order. The prescription pills are usually amphetamine-based drugs that suppress the appetite, but have addictive and far-reaching side effects. I'm sure you're aware of newspaper articles reporting that some of the mail order pills are merely placebos, while others are made of questionable substances that can, in certain people, cause harmful reactions. All we have to do to see the damage such pills cause is to look at the number of high-profile women who have had to check into various clinics around the country to be "dried out" because of addictions, many of which began with diet pills.

These people are looking for an easy fix, an easy way to control their body fat.

Then there are the fad diets. It seems as if we go through periods where there is a fad diet released every few weeks. Low carbohydrates. Grapefruit. High protein. No protein. Turnips and onions. Pasta only. Liquid diets, oatmeal diets, no-dieting diets. The list is endless, and the diets are not scientific.

Now some people hoping to lose weight are having it removed by plastic surgeons: fat is sucked out of the thighs, the buttocks, the cheeks, the upper arms, the ankles, everywhere.

Everyone is looking for the quick and easy—and the "in"—fix.

And do you notice something about all of these methods?

Diet pills. Fad diets. Special diets. Cosmetic surgery.

What do they have in common? They all cost money for something that could be prevented.

There is no great mystery about losing body fat and then keeping it off. Here is the simple formula:

Body Fat = Calories In vs. Calories Out

If you're taking in more calories than you're burning up, you're going to gain weight through stored fat.

That's it. That's the great—and simple—secret behind gaining and maintaining a desired body weight.

The only problem with this simple formula is that it requires some work and dedication.

When you take diet pills to suppress your appetite or when you go on a diet, you eat less.

And often, what you *are* eating while taking diet pills or while on a restrictive diet is food that is not especially good for you, such as junk food and processed food.

Your body requires a certain amount of nutritious foods with adequate vitamins and minerals every day if it is going to maintain good health.

Even if you are mature and sedentary, it is practically impossible to receive all the essential vitamins and minerals you need each day on a diet below 1,400 calories.

What *can* you do to lose excess body fat while also receiving your daily minimums of nutrients? You can eat more!

Whoa! you say. Eat more? But that will put more fat into my body, not less.

You would be right, if we weren't adding the missing element: movement.

Movement in the form of daily aerobic exercise.

What does daily aerobic exercise do?

You remember earlier in this chapter we talked about the metabolic rate and how it is very high in younger children as they are growing and how it slows down as we age? Well, exercise—especially aerobic exercise—stokes the metabolism. Rather than suffering through your adult life with the metabolic rate of an older person, you can stoke your metabolic rate up to a level that puts it at that of a twenty-five-year-old. You recall seventy-year-old Margaret Lee running marathons. You don't for a minute think Margaret has the metabolism of a typical seventy-year-old, do you?

And here's the beauty of exercising on a regular basis: Once you begin to do it regularly, your metabolic rate not only rises while you are exercising, *your metabolic rate stays higher for hours and hours afterward,* which means that besides burning significantly more calories while you are exercising, your body *continues to burn extra calories* for hours and hours afterward.

So, instead of eating 1,400 calories a day, which may not be providing sufficient nourishment (and which could therefore open you up to various sicknesses and diseases), you can eat 2,000 or 2,200 calories a day, receive sufficient vitamins, minerals, and nutrients, and still lose weight, because with daily exercise, you might well be burning 2,500 calories a day.

As an example, if you eat 2,200 calories a day and burn 2,500 calories a day, you are losing 300 calories a day, which means that since there are 3,500 calories in a pound of body fat, each twelve days you'll lose a pound. For quick-fix addicts, that doesn't seem like a lot, but rapid weight loss can be dangerous to your health, and losing one pound every twelve days is a sane and sensible way to lose weight. By this method, you'll lose roughly thirty pounds a year.

So it stands to reason that the more exercise you do, the more calories you burn up—and the more calories you burn up, the faster you will lose weight.

But, that's not all! Besides losing the weight, the exercise will cause you to build muscle tone and muscle strength. You'll look better, you'll feel better, your body will be healthy and more equipped to resist sickness and disease.

And, energy begets energy! This means that your exercising, your trimmed down slimmed down self will be ready to live life to its fullest.

You may be sitting there saying to yourself, "That's all well and good in theory, but I haven't exercised in the last fifty years. That just isn't for me!"

I've spoken to groups of older people for years, and this is usually their sad refrain. "This isn't for me."

What a defeatist attitude! That's not the kind of attitude that gets things done. That's the attitude of someone who has who has given up, who might just as well not get out of bed in the morning.

We have been led to believe that just because we are older, we are frail. That's nonsense! The only thing that makes us frail is if we act frail.

Fortunately, more and more recent research has given me more and more ammunition I can use when I speak to groups of older Americans.

There was an experiment with ninety-year-olds reported in the *Journal of the American Medical Association* in a June 1990 issue. The experiment involved going into a

Boston nursing home and putting six women and four men between eighty-five and ninety-five years of age on an eight-week strength training program. Here's an exact quote from the newspaper story by Thomas H. Maugh II of the Los Angeles *Times* Syndicate:

> Two of the patients who walked with a cane at the beginning of the program can now manage without; one can rise from a chair without using his arms for the first time in years; and five of them walk 50 percent faster. All are more mobile, have better balance, and have suffered fewer falls since the training began.
>
> "The importance of this study is that it shows that, even at a very advanced age, physical frailty is treatable," said Evan Hadley, chief of the geriatric branch at the National Institute of Aging. "This could greatly reduce the need for nursing home admissions by maintaining the mobility of older people and thus their ability to live independently."

It has also been known for some years that regular aerobic exercise contributes to creating denser bones, something of interest to all mature people. Exercise can turn your life around.

If this works with ninety-year-olds, just think what it can do for you!

Eat a good, well-balanced diet and get some daily exercise and you've got the prescription for not only a healthy life beyond fifty, but an incredibly active life. The exercise you take on can—and should—be as simple as a regular walking program, something you already know how to do. (See *Dynastride!*, my walking program, distributed by Penguin Books.)

Go on a "way of life"! It is time to simplify your life, to take life by the scruff of the neck and tell it what you want from it instead of sitting around taking whatever it dishes out.

Don't let life dictate to you. *You* take control. Live life to the fullest, live life the way *you* want to live it.

Eat well, exercise regularly, play well, and be happy.

PART II

A Recipe for Peak Nutrition

Planning a Menu

The second part of this book deals with preparing food to help increase your good health while decreasing your chances of ill health. Chapters 6 through 11 contain recipes that are designed to minimize bad foods and maximize good foods in your daily diet. The recipes are chosen based upon the Peak Nutrition theories we have discussed in the first four chapters.

In this chapter, I'd like to give you some food for thought:

1. How eating habits and lifestyle change as a person ages, and how to keep these changes under control.
2. How to cook creatively for yourself and your friends. Also how to get the most nourishment from your food and the most value for your food dollar, while simplifying your life.
3. How to put together a week's worth of menus based upon the recipes that follow.
4. How to start and keep a food and exercise diary.

This chapter, then, serves as a transition from the theories in the first half of this book to the practical application of the recipes that follow.

YOUR CHANGING FOOD AND LIFESTYLE NEEDS

As we move through life, our nutritional needs change. So do our lifestyles and the way we take in and use food.

We've already discussed the changes in metabolism that accompany us through the phases of our life. As we grow older, unless we do something to keep our body's boiler room (metabolism) active, the fires that sustain us burn down. Consequently, we do not need as much food (calories) as we did when we were younger. Because we are frequently less active, our metabolism is centered on maintenance instead of maintenance *and* growth: Therefore we need less fuel. Unfortunately, we sometimes continue eating the same as we did at half our current age, which only adds to our body weight. Therefore the secret is to remain active while eating only the foods that are good for us.

Besides undergoing changes in our metabolism throughout our life, we also undergo changes in the matter of how we take in our food. When we were children, our food was provided for us by our mothers. When we went to school, we brought our lunch or ate in the cafeteria. Once out on our own, either solo or starting a family, we often learned to cook much as our mothers had cooked before us. While raising our children, meals typically became the central gathering point of all the family members, usually in the early evening.

But, once the children were gone, our cooking habits changed. This is especially true if our mate passed away. Instead of cooking for an army, we were now either cooking for ourselves or for two of us.

However, our lifelong eating habits were still in effect: we continued to eat the same kinds of foods our mothers taught us.

Often people who are widowed no longer like to cook for themselves and lose interest in food. Consequently, some merely nibble instead of eating a well-balanced diet to keep their overall health at its peak and their bones strong.

A person's lifestyle in the later years should be one filled with a zest for life, filled with projects, things to do, places to go, people to see. Too many people reach sixty years of age and wait around for nothing to happen. Unfortunately, they often get what they expected.

Enhance your life with these three things: good food (as fuel), exercise (to keep the body fit), and a will to enjoy both the quantity and the *quality* of life.

COOK CREATIVELY

Many seniors who do not cook for themselves do so for one of two reasons: They are relieved to be rid of the burden of preparing meals once their families are gone, or they are unaware of the importance of nutritious foods—and have not been able to restructure their thinking to make cooking fun.

Let's look at the following six guidelines that may help you eat better while having fun at the same time:

1. Cook in volume. If you have an aversion to cooking because it is too much work for just one or two of you, try this: Cook as though the family *were* still there. Cook in volume. And break the extra food down into meal-size packages, mark them with contents and date, and freeze them. Now when you want to enjoy that meal again, all you need to do is go to the freezer and thaw and reheat it or microwave it. There are many packages and containers available to conveniently freeze and store food.

This practice is one that I call cooking-for-an-army. It works especially well when you're cooking soups or spaghetti sauce or baking muffins. Make your cooking-for-an-army an enjoyable project. Put on some good music and then cook up a storm. Serve a meal from what you've just cooked, and freeze the rest. *Voilà!* You have just saved yourself a great deal of time down the line. And don't forget that with some foods, they also taste better the second time around.

2. Form cooking/eating groups. A wonderfully social way to eat well most nights of the week is to put together a cooking/eating group. Such a group can consist of as few as two people or as many as five or six. Each person signs up to take a specific night of the week, and the group gathers at that person's house that night for dinner. No, you don't burden that one person with all the work. The host or hostess is responsible for the entrée and the rest of the group is responsible for everything else: salad, bread, appetizer, vegetables, dessert, etc. It is a wonderfully social, communal way of eating and keeping in contact with good friends.

You can also occasionally have theme nights. Perhaps on the first Wednesday of each month you can have a lean beef night. Or a "fun with turkey" night. Or how about a meatless night? You'd be surprised how delicious a meatless meal can be with a little planning. Or you can have ethnic nights: South of the Border Night, Oriental Night, Greek Night, Italian Night, Soul Food Night, Creole Night. Be creative, but make certain to cook nutritiously. Skip the Liver and Onions Nights.

3. Don't fight routine. Because of the busy, hectic life I've chosen to lead, I'm not into much of a routine. But I also know that for many people it is a comforting anchor in life to have a routine of some sort.

I wholeheartedly endorse trying new things, especially when it involves breaking old habits in order to replace them with new habits that lead to more nutritious eating.

One way is to develop a routine where you put together a logical, nutritious week-long menu based upon the recipes that come later in this book. (In fact, to help you in that regard, later in this chapter I've put together a week-long menu.) If you like them, introduce them into your menus.

4. Keep the ingredients handy. One thing that discourages me from getting really psyched up to cook is to pull out recipes and pots and pans and then find that I don't have some of the ingredients handy. This is especially inconvenient because we live several miles from town.

As a result, I now make sure that I keep a good supply of spices and herbs handy, as well as things that I normally use in cooking.

Also, before I go shopping I try to figure out just what I'm going to cook, then I pull out the recipes and either copy down what I'm going to need from the store or else take the recipes with me (see next section). Once I work up a head of steam for cooking, I don't want to be deflated by finding that I don't have what I need handy.

5. Simplify your cooking. Often when we cook, we don't take the time to organize ourselves and we consequently have too many pots and pans and ingredients all over the kitchen. It looks like a disaster area. Take time to organize. Put out all the ingredients you are going to use. If you run out of an ingredient, keep a pad and pencil handy to write it down right away. My sister-in-law Pat keeps a blackboard in her kitchen by the telephone, and when she wants to remember something she writes it down immediately. Therefore she is always on top of things. Another little hint to keep your kitchen more organized is to wash the cooking dishes and utensils as soon as you are finished using them. Your kitchen will always look neat and cooking won't be so laborious.

Cookbooks can also cause problems. They fall over, pages flop over and they get soiled. If you have this problem, put your cookbook in a book holder and cover the page and book with plastic wrap so that any spills can be wiped off. You can buy plastic adjustable holders that your cookbook will fit into, thereby keeping it clean while the page you want is held open for you.

You can also buy 3x5-inch plastic recipe holders into which you can slide recipe cards to keep them from getting soiled. Another idea is to mount them into photo albums. If you have trouble reading small print on a 3x5 card, use one of the larger 4x6 cards available at stationery stores.

And don't stop with the recipes in this book. Some of the major supermarkets and health food stores issue recipe cards with an eye toward nutritious meals—and some of them are printed on special card stock that can be wiped clean after using.

6. Be resourceful. Recipes are not written in stone. Be creative with them by adding your own twists and changing the ingredients.

When I decided I no longer wanted to be a junk food junkie, the first thing I did was to broil everything I used to fry. The second change I made was to make some healthful cookies for the children. In those days there were very few health food cookbooks, so I took an oatmeal cookie recipe and substituted oil for the butter, honey for the sugar, and whole wheat flour for white flour. I added a few walnuts and raisins and—*Voila!*—all the kids in the neighborhood loved them.

My writing partner, Rich Benyo, some years ago took a simple whole wheat bread recipe and experimented with it, removing the salt, adding raisins and nuts and nutmeg, until he was able to win a ribbon at the Napa Valley County Fair.

Use the recipes as a starting point. Not all recipes will be to your taste, but with a little creative change here or there, you can *make* them to your taste. Do you like nutmeg? If an apple pie recipe says add 1 teaspoon nutmeg, add more if you like more. Remember that as we age our taste buds don't work as well. Sometimes a spice or an herb needs to be doubled for it to work well. Also, why not sprinkle a handful of raisins over your apple pie before you put the top crust over it? Trust yourself. Go with your instincts. You have nobody to please but yourself. Let your creative side show. Experiment on yourself, and when you make creative changes that work, you can present your very own creation at your next meal with friends. They'll be *so* impressed.

A WEEK'S WORTH OF MEALS

What comes next is a week's menu put together from the recipes in the chapters that follow. It is used as an example of how you can plan out recipes for a week. Once you've planned those menus, you don't have to think about what you are going to eat for the rest of the week. It's all written down, and all you need do is follow your own outline.

Here are some suggestions for menu planning starting with Monday and ending with the Sunday meal. You might want to make more on Sunday so that you can incorporate leftovers into the menu for the following week. You might also like to combine breakfast and lunch into a brunch on Sunday.

|●| *Monday: breakfast*
Banana toast
Favorite juice
Herbal tea

|●| *Monday: lunch*
Jack's blender soup

|●| *Monday: dinner*
Jack's chop-chop
I slice easy French bread
Choose a dessert from chapter 9

|●| *Tuesday: breakfast*
Almond fig compote
Choice of muffins from chapter 6
Herbal tea

|●| *Tuesday: lunch*
Jon's tempting tuna salad
Water

|●| *Tuesday: dinner*
Wheat chili
Thyme carrots
Choose a dessert from chapter 9

|●| *Wednesday: breakfast*
Grains and goodies

|●| *Wednesday: lunch*
Today's healthy corn chowder

|●| *Wednesday: dinner*
Elaine's stuffed cabbage

|●| *Thursday: breakfast*
Bragg's pep health drink

|●| *Thursday: lunch*
Crustless chard quiche

|●| *Thursday: dinner*
Luscious lemon chicken
Squash medley
Potatoes LaLanne

⦿ *Friday: breakfast*
Brown rice cereal

⦿ *Friday: lunch*
Cheryl's sunflower slaw
1 slice Mother's whole wheat

⦿ *Friday: dinner*
Mollie's classic poached salmon or
broiled whitefish
Brown and wild rice casserole

⦿ *Saturday: breakfast*
Breakfast burritos or
Jack's egg white omelet
Fresh fruit

⦿ *Saturday: lunch*
Tofu patty

⦿ *Saturday: dinner*
Paella or
California cioppino
1 slice easy French bread

⦿ *Sunday: brunch*
Quickie applesauce or
Cranberry blush
Buttermilk pancakes

⦿ *Sunday: dinner*
Roast stuffed leg of lamb
Ratatouille

YOUR PEAK NUTRITION AND FITNESS DIARY

One of the main ingredients in my previous three books was keeping a diary of your fitness achievements. In this book, keeping a diary is almost essential. It's a great way to check on your eating habits, fitness activities, and your life in general. It will help you record your progress while you improve your eating habits and get in some exercise. As you progress, your periodic medical checkups should begin to improve, along with your body's profile. Don't expect immediate results, but *do* expect gradual improvements.

Unlike previous diary pages from my other books, *Fitness After 50, Dynastride!* and *The Fitness After 50 Workout,* this one is special. For this book I've put together a diary

MY PEAK NUTRITION & FITNESS DAILY DIARY

DATE	MONTH	YEAR	DAY OF WEEK	RESTING PULSE RATE AT RISING

BREAKFAST
_____
_____
_____
_____
_____
_____
_____
_____
_____

LUNCH
_____
_____
_____
_____
_____
_____
_____
_____
_____

DINNER
_____
_____
_____
_____
_____
_____
_____

SNACKS
_____
_____
_____
_____
_____
_____

WATER   1   2   3   4   5   6   7   8   9   10   11   12   GLASSES

THINGS TO DO/THINGS I DID

7 a.m. _____	3 p.m. _____
8 a.m. _____	4 p.m. _____
9 a.m. _____	5 p.m. _____
10 a.m. _____	6 p.m. _____
11 a.m. _____	7 p.m. _____
noon _____	8 p.m. _____
1 p.m. _____	9 p.m. _____
2 p.m _____	10 p.m. _____

BODY PROFILE

Body Weight _____   Hips in Inches _____
Chest in inches _____   Thigh in Inches   (left)   (right) _____
Waist in inches _____   Upper arms in inches   (left)   (right) _____

FITNESS   **COMMENTS:**

Type of Activity _____   _____
Duration of Activity _____ _____
Perceived Effort _____   _____

REFLECTIONS ON MY DAY

_____   _____
_____   _____
_____   _____
_____   _____
_____   _____
_____   _____
_____   _____
_____   _____
_____   _____
_____   _____
_____   _____
_____   _____
_____   _____

that is designed to devote an entire page to each day. So you can make longer entries, and completely record your day's fitness and health activities, you may want to make copies of these pages as needed, punch them, and put them into a three-ring binder. Here's what you'll find on each diary page:

Date: On this line, write in today's date, the month, the year, and the day of the week.

Resting pulse rate at rising. A measure of your fitness is your pulse rate first thing in the morning. Take your pulse rate while still in bed, using the pulse point at either the neck or the wrist. As you become healthier and more fit, your pulse rate will drop, indicating that your heart is working more efficiently.

Food diary. In these sections, keep track of *everything* you ate during the day. The three primary meals are easy to keep track of, but I've also added a Snacks column, which is a catchall for anything you eat between meals or after the dinner meal. Everything you put into your mouth during the day should go here. At the bottom of this section is a section for water; this is where you can keep track of the number of glasses of water you drink during the day. Remember! Attempt to drink eight glasses a day.

Things to do. In this section, keep track of the things you have to do for the day. This works perfectly as a reference in case you need to look back to check what you did at this time last week or last year. It also serves as a good reminder of appointments for the day.

Body profile. As you become healthier and more fit, the shape of your body will change. Keep track of your body's statistics every day: body weight, chest measurement, waist measurement, hips measurement, measurement of thighs, and measurement of the upper arm. Once you've been on a program of good eating and mild fitness for three to four months, compare your body measurements with what they were when you started. The changes will not come rapidly, but by pacing yourself, they *will* come, and once they are there, they will stay.

Fitness diary. In this section, keep track of the type of fitness activity in which you've engaged during the day. Did you go for a walk? Did you join an exercise class? Did you go bicycling? Virtually *any* physical activity will help round out your health. In the far right space, keep track of how you felt during the workout, if you enjoyed it, how you felt afterward, etc.

Reflections on my day. This is where you can reflect on the day you have just had. This is the space where you can write anything you want. What did you think about during the day? Did you finish that book you were reading? Was it any good? Did you write a letter or two? Did you think about planning a trip? Did you watch your favorite soap opera this afternoon? This is the space where you can put your thoughts, your feelings, your aspirations. You needn't write a book every day. But at least write something.

ABOUT THE RECIPES THAT FOLLOW

Over the years, I've collected the following recipes from friends, neighbors, and acquaintances. I appreciate the willingness of so many people to share their secrets of creating nutritious and appetizing meals. All recipes not credited to an individual or an organization are from the kitchens of Elaine and Jack LaLanne.

Nutritional information that accompanies the recipes in chapters 6 through 11 is calibrated by nutritional computer based upon the smallest number of servings if there is a range, i.e., serves 2 to 3, on the smaller amount of an ingredient where a range is given, i.e., 2 to 2 1/2 cups, and does not include optional ingredients when such ingredients are given.

If you have special dietary needs or requirements due to an existing medical condition, consult your physician before trying new recipes.

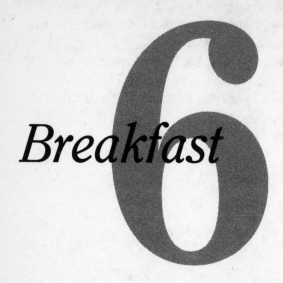

Breakfast

▣ Elaine's Wheat Germ Muffins

1 cup whole wheat flour (sifted)
2 1/2 tsps baking powder with a pinch of salt
1/4 cup bran
1 cup raw wheat germ
2/3 cup skim milk
1 egg
1/4 cup safflower oil
1/4 cup honey
1/2 cup raisins or 1/2 cup chopped apples

1. Sift whole wheat flour, baking powder, and salt together and then add other ingredients. Mix together. Spoon into muffin papers.
2. Bake in a preheated oven at 400 degrees for 25 minutes.

Variations:

1. Substitute molasses for honey. Substitute buttermilk for skim milk.
2. Substitute orange or apple juice for milk and add 2 tablespoons orange peel.

YIELDS: 1 DOZEN MUFFINS

Nutritional breakdown: 5 grams protein, 24 grams carbohydrate, 6 grams fat*
Serving: 1 muffin
Calories per serving: 160

*Note: Nutritional breakdown is for *entire* recipe.

LaLanne Banana Muffins

I cup honey
1/2 cup safflower oil
3 egg whites, or 2 whole eggs, slightly
  beaten
3 large ripe bananas, mashed (I 1/2 cups)
1/2 tsp lemon juice (optional)
2 cups whole wheat pastry flour
I tsp baking soda
I tsp vanilla extract
I cup chopped nuts (coarse)
1/4 cup wheat germ or safflower seeds
  (optional)

1. Combine honey and oil; add eggs, mashed bananas, and lemon juice.
2. Sift flour and baking soda together and stir into banana mixture. Add vanilla, nuts, and wheat germ.
3. Bake in a preheated oven at 350 degrees for 35 to 45 minutes in a paper-lined or slightly oiled muffin pan. May also be made in a standard loaf pan (oiled with vegetable spray).

YIELDS: 2 DOZEN MUFFINS

Nutritional breakdown: 4 grams protein, 24 grams carbohydrate, 8 grams fat
Serving portion: I muffin
Calories per serving: 175
Recipe courtesy Dr. Yvonne LaLanne-Rubenstein

No, No-No Muffins *(no salt, sugar, or oil)*

2 large ripe bananas, or I cup coarsely
  chopped apples
3 egg whites, or 2 large eggs
I (6 oz) can undiluted juice concentrate
  (orange, apple, or pineapple)
2 cups unbleached or whole wheat flour
I tsp baking soda
3 tsps baking powder
I tsp cinnamon
I tsp pumpkin pie spice (or use 1/4 tsp each
  of nutmeg, ginger, clove, allspice)
1/3 cup raisins
1/3 cup chopped nuts (optional)

1. Preheat oven to 350 degrees.
2. Mash bananas in a large mixing bowl.
3. Add eggs and undiluted juice. Beat until fluffy.
4. Mix flour, baking soda, baking powder, and spices in a separate bowl; add to banana mixture. Stir in raisins and nuts.
5. Bake in 16 to 18 muffin cups or one loaf pan. Because no shortening is used in the batter, it is necessary to use nonstick cooking spray in pans and inside paper cups or inside loaf pan.
6. Bake approximately 20 minutes, or until knife inserted in center comes out clean.

YIELDS: I 1/2 DOZEN MUFFINS

Nutritional breakdown: 6 grams protein, 38 grams carbohydrate, 0 grams fat
Serving portion: 2 muffins
Calories per serving: 174

Fruitful Muffins

1 cup Quaker Oats (quick or old-fashioned,
  uncooked)
1 cup unbleached flour
1 tbsp baking powder
1/2 tsp cinnamon
1 cup skim milk
1/2 cup mashed ripe banana (about 1 large)
1/2 cup raisins
1/4 cup vegetable oil
1/4 cup firmly packed brown sugar
1 egg white

1. Heat oven to 400 degrees.
2. Line 12 medium muffin cups with paper baking cups. Combine oats, flour, baking powder, and cinnamon. Combine remaining ingredients and add to flour mixture; mix just until dry ingredients are moistened. Fill prepared muffin cups three-quarters full. Bake 20 to 25 minutes, or until golden brown.

Variation:

Substitute 1/2 cup chopped apricots, dates, or prunes for raisins.

YIELDS: 1 DOZEN MUFFINS

Nutritional breakdown: 3 grams protein, 240 grams carbohydrate, 5 grams fat
Serving portion: 1 muffin
Calories per serving: 160
Recipe courtesy Quaker Oats Company

Oat-Berry Muffins

1 cup oat flour
1 tsp baking soda
1/4 tsp salt
3/4 cup plain nonfat yogurt
1/3 cup honey
1 egg
2 tbsps vegetable oil
3/4 cup blueberries

Topping:

1 tbsp quick oats
1/2 tsp cinnamon
1 tsp natural fructose

1. Sift together flour, baking soda, and salt; set aside.
2. Combine yogurt, honey, egg, and oil.
3. Add dry ingredients and stir well to combine.
4. Gently fold in blueberries.
5. Scoop batter into paper-lined muffin cups.
6. Top with cinnamon-oat mixture.
7. Bake at 350 degrees for approximately 30 minutes, or until a toothpick comes out clean.

YIELDS: 8 LARGE MUFFINS

Nutritional breakdown: 4 grams protein, 28 grams carbohydrate, 4 grams fat
Serving portion: 1 muffin
Calories per serving: 161

Brown Rice Cereal

4 oz brown rice, cooked

Top with your favorite:

1/4 cup skim milk
1/4 cup Quickie Applesauce (page 78)
2 tbsps raisins
1 tbsp wheat germ

Variation:

Use cooked wheat berries (whole grain wheat) instead of rice.

YIELDS: 1 SERVING

Nutritional breakdown: 8 grams protein, 65 grams carbohydrate, 2 grams fat
Serving portion: 1 bowl
Calories per serving: 298

 # Grains and Goodies

1/3 cup bulgur or fortified oat flake cereal
1/2 cup cornmeal
3 oz dried fruit bits or raisins
1/4 cup toasted almond slivers
Cinnamon to taste
2 cups boiling water

1. Combine grains, fruit, nuts, and cinnamon with the boiling water in an uncovered pot; stir slowly.
2. Return to a boil and lower to simmer for 10 to 15 minutes, or until ingredients reach desired consistency.

YIELDS: 2 CUPS

Nutritional breakdown: 4 grams protein, 31 grams carbohydrate, 4 grams fat
Serving portion: 1/2 cup
Calories per serving: 166

Unsweetened applesauce may be substituted for oil in muffin recipes—if you use a slightly larger amount than that called for.

Delicious Granola

5 cups rolled oats
1 cup wheat germ
1 cup soy flour
1 cup sunflower seeds
1 cup chopped almonds
1 cup powdered milk
1/2 cup honey
1/2 cup safflower oil
10 dried dates
10 dried prunes

1. Combine dry ingredients.
2. In a separate bowl, combine the honey and oil. Pour over dry ingredients. Mix well and spread on two large cookie sheets.
3. Bake at 275 degrees for about 40 minutes.
4. Check after 20 minutes. It should be slightly brown to bring out the flavor.
5. Cut up the pitted dates and prunes and add to cereal. Store in refrigerator.

YIELDS: 12 CUPS

Nutritional breakdown: 9 grams protein, 26 grams carbohydrate, 13 grams fat
Serving portion: 1/2 cup
Calories per serving: 240

Granola Bars

1/4 cup raw honey
1/2 cup raw unsalted peanut butter
1 tbsp margarine or safflower oil
1 tsp vanilla extract
2 cups granola

1. Preheat oven to 350 degrees.
2. Mix all the ingredients together and spread in an 8-inch-square Pyrex pan, approximately 1/2 inch thick.
3. You may vary these bars by adding raisins, nuts, dates, or sunflower seeds.
4. Bake approximately 10 minutes.
5. Allow to cool and cut into 2-inch squares.

YIELDS: 16 SQUARES

Nutritional breakdown: 3 grams protein, 14 grams carbohydrate, 5 grams fat
Serving portion: 1 square
Calories per serving: 110

Buttermilk Pancakes

1 tbsp safflower oil
3 egg whites, or 2 eggs
3/4 cup buttermilk (if you do not have
  buttermilk, substitute 3/4 cup skim milk
  and 2 tsps lemon juice or vinegar)
1 tsp baking soda, dissolved in 1/4 cup warm
  water
1 tsp baking powder
1/2 tsp salt
1/4 cup cornmeal

1. Preheat griddle to correct pancake temperature.
2. Whip eggs until fluffy, beat in buttermilk, oil and baking soda. Add dry ingredients to liquid mixture until well blended.
3. Bake on oiled griddle, turning when bottom is golden brown.
4. Top with Quickie Applesauce (page 78) or pure maple syrup (optional).

YIELDS: 2 SERVINGS

Nutritional breakdown: 10 grams protein, 19 grams carbohydrate, 8 grams fat
Serving portion: 1/2 recipe
Calories per serving: 188

 # *High-Protein Pancakes*

6 egg whites, or 4 eggs
1 cup low-fat cottage cheese
2 tbsps safflower oil
1/2 cup oatmeal (or 1/4 cup wheat germ and
  1/4 cup oatmeal)
1/4 tsp salt

1. Place all ingredients in a blender and mix thoroughly.
2. Drop by tablespoons onto a hot frying pan or griddle oiled with polyunsaturated oil.

YIELDS: 4 SERVINGS

Nutritional breakdown: 14 grams protein, 5 grams carbohydrate, 15 grams fat
Serving portion: 1/4 batter
Calories per serving: 208

For a delicious toast or pancake spread, puree fresh fruit or berries in a blender. You can keep the spread handy in a covered container in the refrigerator. Rehydrated dried fruit also works well.

Blintzes

4 egg whites, or 3 eggs
1 cup skim milk or water
1/2 tsp salt
3 tbsps safflower oil
3/4 cup sifted unbleached flour

1. Beat eggs, skim milk, salt, and 2 tablespoons of the oil together. Stir in flour.
2. Heat the remaining 1 tablespoon safflower oil in a 6-inch skillet.
3. Pour about 2 tablespoons of the batter into it, tilting the pan to coat the bottom. Use just enough batter to make a very thin pancake. Let the bottom brown, then carefully turn out onto a napkin, browned side up. Repeat until all the batter is used.
4. Fill blintzes with Quickie Applesauce (page 78) and roll up for serving.

YIELDS: 3 SERVINGS

Nutritional breakdown: 11 grams protein, 27 grams carbohydrate, 14 grams fat
Serving portion: 1/3 blintz batter
Calories per serving (not including filling): 286

Old-Fashioned Oat Bran Pancakes

Egg substitute for 1 egg
2 egg whites
1 cup skim milk
3 tbsps corn oil
8 oz plain low-fat yogurt
1/4 cup honey
1 tbsp vanilla extract
1 1/4 cups unsifted flour
1/2 cup fine oat or wheat bran
1 tsp baking powder
1 tsp baking soda
1/4 tsp salt

1. In a large bowl, beat egg substitute and egg whites with a wire whisk until frothy.
2. Beat in milk, corn oil, yogurt, honey, and vanilla until blended. Add flour, bran, baking powder, baking soda, and salt; beat until blended.
3. For each pancake, spoon 3 tablespoons batter onto a hot, lightly greased griddle. Cook over medium heat 4 minutes, turning once, or until browned. If desired, serve with sliced fruit.

YIELDS: 24 (4-INCH) PANCAKES

Nutritional breakdown: 8 grams protein, 31 grams carbohydrate, 6 grams fat
Serving portion: 3 pancakes
Calories per serving: 210
Recipe courtesy Mazola corn oil

Norwegian Waffles

3 egg whites, or 2 eggs
1/4 cup honey
1 1/2 cups whole wheat flour
1 1/2 tsps baking powder
1 tsp baking soda
1/2 tsp salt
1/4 tsp ground cardamom
2 cups buttermilk
2 tbsps safflower oil

1. Beat eggs and honey until light and creamy. Mix all dry ingredients and add them to the honey mixture alternately with the buttermilk. Add oil.
2. Cook waffles in a waffle iron.
3. Serve hot or cold with applesauce or any fresh fruit.

YIELDS: 4 WAFFLES

Nutritional breakdown: 13 grams protein, 55 grams carbohydrate, 12 grams fat
Serving portion: 1 waffle
Calories per serving: 365
Recipe courtesy Betty Ann Quist

Breakfast Burritos

1 tbsp olive oil
1 small green or red bell pepper, or both, chopped fine
1 boiled potato with skin, chopped coarse
3 egg whites, beaten
1 tbsp chopped onion (optional)
2 whole wheat tortillas

1. Preheat a skillet with 1 tablespoon oil or more, as needed. Sauté peppers and onions, then add potatoes and sauté slightly.
2. Add eggs and stir until desired consistency.
3. Roll up in warmed whole wheat tortillas and add salsa, if desired.

YIELDS: 2 BURRITOS

Nutritional breakdown: 9 grams protein, 33 grams carbohydrate, 9 grams fat
Serving portion: 1 burrito
Calories per serving: 246

Jack's Egg White Omelet

3 to 4 egg whites
1 tbsp water
Pinch of vegetable salt and pepper to taste
1 tsp fresh basil
2 tbsps chopped green or red bell pepper
2 tbsps chopped fresh tomato

1. Lightly coat an omelet pan with safflower oil.
2. Blend eggs, water, and salt and pepper. Pour into heated pan, turning pan to allow egg to run under cooked portion. When mixture is almost set, add basil, bell pepper, and fresh tomato. Using a spatula, carefully flip half of omelet over filling.

YIELDS: 1 OMELET

Nutritional breakdown: 13 grams protein, 9 grams carbohydrate, 0 grams fat
Serving portion: 1
Calories per serving: 92

 # *Bragg's Pep Health Drink*

Juice of 2 to 3 oranges (fresh) or
  unsweetened pineapple juice, or 1 glass
  distilled water
1 tsp raw wheat germ
1 tsp brewer's yeast
1 tbsp raw oat bran
1 tbsp lecithin granules
1/2 tsp vitamin C powder
1/3 tsp pure pectin powder
1/2 ripe banana
1/2 tsp honey
1 tbsp soy protein powder
1/2 tsp raisins
1 tsp raw sunflower or pumpkin seeds

Mix all ingredients in a blender, adding 1 ice cube if desired chilled.

YIELDS: 2 SERVINGS

Nutritional breakdown: 4 grams protein, 24 grams carbohydrate, 10 grams fat
Serving portion: 1/2 contents
Calories per serving: 200
Recipe courtesy Patricia Bragg

Mock Milk

1 cup blanched almonds
4 tsps honey
2 cups water
1 cup ice cubes

Process almonds in a blender until mealy. Add water, ice cubes, and honey; blend. May be served strained if desired.

YIELDS: 1 QUART

Nutritional breakdown: 6.5 grams protein, 30 grams carbohydrate, 17 grams fat
Serving portion: 1 cup
Calories per serving: 279
(If not used as main source of calories for breakfast, cut recipe portion in half.)

Norwegian Frukt-Suppe (Fruit Soup)

3 cups dried diced mixed fruit
2 cups seeded and diced apples
1/2 cup honey
2 1/2 cups boiling water
1 stick cinnamon
1/4 tsp salt
1/2 cup quick-cooking tapioca
2 cups white grape juice
1 tbsp vinegar or lemon juice

1. Combine all ingredients except grape juice and vinegar. Bring to a boil. Reduce heat. Cover and simmer, stirring frequently.
2. When tapioca is clear, add juice and vinegar and return to a boil. Serve hot or cold for breakfast or as a dessert.

YIELDS: 8 CUPS

Nutritional breakdown: 1 gram protein, 37 grams carbohydrate, 0 grams fat
Serving portion: 1/2 cup
Calories per serving: 143
Recipe courtesy Betty Ann Quist

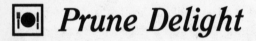 Quickie Applesauce

2 to 3 apples
1/2 cup water
Honey or pure maple syrup to taste
1 tsp lemon juice
Dash of cinnamon

1. Wash, quarter, and core apples.
2. Place all ingredients except cinnamon in a blender or food processor. Process so that apples remain chunky.
3. Pour into a saucepan and cook until bubbly.
4. Add cinnamon and serve. Delicious over oatmeal, whole grain toast, or whole grain dry cereals.

YIELDS: 2 CUPS

Nutritional breakdown: 0 grams protein, 15 grams carbohydrate, 0 grams fat
Serving portion: 1/2 cup
Calories per serving: 60
Recipe courtesy Patricia LaLanne

Prune Delight

20 large prunes (dried)
1/2 cup honey
2 tsps lemon juice
6 egg whites

1. Cook prunes well. Stone and chop.
2. Add honey and lemon juice.
3. Beat egg whites until they hold a point. Fold into prune mixture, then spoon into a casserole and place in a pan of hot water. Bake for about 40 minutes in a 325-degree oven. Serve warm or cold.
4. Optional: sprinkle lightly with granola.

YIELDS: 6 SERVINGS

Nutritional breakdown: 3 grams protein, 43 grams carbohydrate, 0 grams fat
Serving portion: 1/6 recipe
Calories per serving: 170
Recipe courtesy Elaine's mother, Betty S. Rorem

Cranberry Blush

1 cup plain low-fat yogurt
1 cup cranberry juice
2 to 3 tbsps nuts (optional)

1. Mix all ingredients well.
2. Serve as a topping on fresh fruit, whole grain toast, pancakes, or waffles.

YIELDS: 2 CUPS

Nutritional breakdown: 2 grams protein, 7 grams carbohydrate, 2 grams fat
Serving portion: 1/4 cup
Calories per serving: 52
Recipe courtesy Connie Haines

 # *Banana Toast*

1/2 to 1 whole banana
1 egg
Mace, nutmeg, cinnamon to taste
1 slice whole grain bread

1. Put banana in a blender or mash.
2. Add egg and spices. Mix well.
3. Dip slice of bread in mixture and brown slightly on each side in a nonstick pan or griddle as you would French toast.

YIELDS: 1 SERVING

Nutritional breakdown: 7 grams protein, 33 grams carbohydrate, 2 grams fat
Serving portion: 1 slice
Calories per serving: 163

Dried fruit can be rehydrated by soaking it in warm apple or orange juice.

7

Lunch, Soups, Salads, and Salad Dressings

 ## *Basic Salad Dressing*

This basic salad dressing will be used with various lunch salads that follow.

1/3 to 1/2 cup olive oil
1/4 cup red wine vinegar
1 tsp garlic powder seasoned with parsley
1 tsp vegetable salt
1 tsp lemon pepper
1 tbsp water

1. Combine all ingredients in a blender and purée until creamy.
2. Adjust seasoning to taste.

YIELDS: 1 CUP

Nutritional breakdown: 0 grams protein, 0 grams carbohydrate, 5 grams fat
Serving portion: 1 tbsp
Calories per serving: 44

Oil your measuring cup before measuring honey for recipes. It allows the honey to slide out easily.

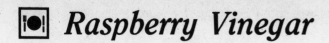 Raspberry Vinegar

1 (16-oz) pkg frozen raspberries
3 cups white vinegar
2 tbsps honey

1. Combine all ingredients in a saucepan and bring to a boil.
2. Remove from heat and allow to cool.
3. Pour liquid through a strainer into a bottle.

YIELDS: 4 CUPS

Nutritional breakdown: 0 grams protein, 1 gram carbohydrate, 0 grams fat
Serving portion: 1 tablespoon
Calories per serving: 4
Recipe courtesy Giselle Ganes

Herb Salad Dressing

1/3 cup white wine vinegar
1 tsp dried parsley flakes
1/2 tsp dried thyme
1/2 tsp dried tarragon
1 garlic clove, minced
1 cup corn oil
1 tbsp chopped onion
1 tsp dry mustard
1/2 tsp salt

1. Combine all ingredients in a container with a tight cover.
2. Shake well and chill.
3. Shake before serving.

YIELDS: 1 1/3 CUPS

Nutritional breakdown: 0 grams protein, 0 grams carbohydrate, 10 grams fat
Serving portion: 1 tablespoon
Calories per serving: 88
Recipe courtesy Mazola corn oil

Oriental Salad Dressing

1/4 cup oriental sesame oil
1/4 cup seasoned rice vinegar

1. Combine both ingredients in a container with a tight cover.
2. Shake well and chill.
3. Shake before serving.

YIELDS: 1/2 CUP

Nutritional breakdown: 0 grams protein, 0 grams carbohydrate, 3 grams fat
Serving portion: 1 tablespoon
Calories per serving: 60

 # Bean Sprout Salad

2 cups fresh bean sprouts
1/2 cup thinly sliced celery
1/2 cup thinly sliced radishes
2 green onions, sliced
1/2 cup carrots
4 tbsps Oriental Salad Dressing (see preceding recipe)

1. Mix together salad ingredients.
2. Shake salad dressing well and pour over salad.

YIELDS: 3 1/2 CUPS

Nutritional breakdown: 9 grams protein, 28 grams carbohydrate, 5 grams fat
Serving portion: 1/2 cup
Calories per serving: 164

Pasta Vegetarian

4 oz uncooked salad pasta
1/2 cup sliced mushrooms
1/2 cup broccoli florets
1/4 cup diced red or green bell peppers or pimiento
1/4 diced red onion
1 medium tomato, diced
1/4 cup diced celery
1/4 cup chopped zucchini
1/4 cup Basic Salad Dressing (page 80)

1. Cook pasta until al dente. Drain and rinse.
2. Combine all salad ingredients in a large bowl. Gently toss with dressing. Chill.

Variation:

Add diced chicken or turkey.

YIELDS: 4 CUPS

Nutritional breakdown: 3 grams protein, 14 grams carbohydrate, 17 grams fat
Serving portion: 1 cup
Calories per serving: 230

Jon's Tempting Tuna Salad

1 (6 1/2-oz) can water-packed tuna
1 (7- to 8-oz) can garbanzo beans, drained
1/2 sweet red pepper (cut into strips)
1/2 green bell pepper (cut into strips)
1/2 cup red onion rings

1. Mix ingredients and serve on a bed of shredded lettuce.
2. Can be garnished with cucumber rounds, bean sprouts, and/or carrot curls.
3. Drizzle with Basic Salad Dressing (page 80) if desired.

YIELDS: 2 SERVINGS

Nutritional breakdown: 31 grams protein, 24 grams carbohydrate, 5 grams fat
Serving portion: 1 1/2 cups
Calories per serving: 262
Recipe courtesy Jon Allen LaLanne

 # Cheryl's Sunflower Slaw

1 1/2 cups shredded cabbage
1 cup shredded carrots
1/2 cup plain low-fat yogurt
2 tbsps sunflower seeds
2 tbsps raisins
3/4 tsp red wine vinegar
1/8 tsp paprika
Sprinkle of garlic

Combine all ingredients and mix well.

YIELDS: 6 SERVINGS

Nutritional breakdown: 2 grams protein, 7.5 grams carbohydrate, 2 grams fat
Serving portion: 1/2 cup
Calories per serving: 52
Recipe courtesy Living Lean by Choosing More, *by Cheryl Jennings-Sauer, MA, RD, LD (Taylor Publishing, 1989)*

 # Kiwi, Orange, and Banana Salad

1 kiwi
1 orange
1 banana

1. Peel and slice kiwi, banana, and orange.
2. Arrange alternately on lettuce bed.

YIELDS: 2 SERVINGS

Nutritional breakdown: 1.5 grams protein, 27 grams carbohydrate, 0 grams fat
Serving portion: 1/2 recipe
Calories per serving: 107

Chinese Chicken Salad

2 cups rice sticks
1/2 head iceberg lettuce, shredded
1/2 head romaine or red lettuce, shredded
3 half chicken breasts, cooked and shredded
1 small bunch green onions, chopped
1/2 cup Oriental Salad Dressing (page 82)

1. Heat rice sticks in hot oil until they puff up. Sizzle a few strands at a time. Do not brown. Drain on paper towels.
2. Mix all ingredients together with dressing and serve immediately.

YIELDS: 4 LARGE SERVINGS

Nutritional breakdown: 23 grams protein, 7 grams carbohydrate, 17 grams fat
Serving portion: 1/4 recipe
Calories per serving: 415
Recipe courtesy Giselle Ganes

 # Energy Salad

1 cup bulgur, fine grind
1 bunch parsley, chopped fine
1 medium tomato, chopped fine
2 to 3 green onions, chopped fine
Season to taste: salt, 1 or 2 mint leaves, lemon juice, safflower oil

1. Soak bulgur in warm water for approximately 1/2 hour. Squeeze dry.
2. Add chopped parsley, tomato, and onions. Season.
3. Serve on lettuce leaf or stuff into tomato.

YIELDS: 2 SERVINGS

Nutritional breakdown: 8 grams protein, 73 grams carbohydrate, 1 gram fat
Serving portion: 1/2 recipe
Calories per serving: 330

Salad of Green and Gold

1/2 avocado
1 large ripe papaya
1 small red onion, cut into rings
2 tbsps chopped fresh mint (optional)
1/4 cup olive oil
2 tbsps Raspberry Vinegar (page 81)
2 cups shredded romaine lettuce

1. Cut avocado and papaya with melon baller, then mix with onion and mint.
2. Combine oil and vinegar and add to mix.
3. Marinate for 1 hour at room temperature.
4. Arrange on lettuce and garnish with mint leaves.

YIELDS: 3 SERVINGS

Nutritional breakdown: 2 grams protein, 8 grams carbohydrate, 24 grams fat
Serving portion: 1/3 recipe
Calories per serving: 234
Recipe courtesy Lucy Thomas, Louisiana Pacific Corp.

 Jack's Blender Soup

1 (16-oz) can chicken broth or 2 cups homemade chicken stock
1 can or 2 cups water
1 garlic clove
1 carrot, chopped
1/2 zucchini, chopped
1 small green bell pepper, chopped
1 celery rib, chopped
1/2 cup chopped onion

1. Mix all the ingredients in a blender. (You may substitute for the above vegetables any you have sitting in your refrigerator waiting to be used.)
2. Pour into a saucepan and bring to a boil. Remove from heat and serve.
3. For cream soup, add 1/2 cup low-fat yogurt and 1 teaspoon dill.

YIELDS: 2 SERVINGS

Nutritional breakdown: 7 grams protein, 12 grams carbohydrate, 2 grams fat
Serving portion: 1/2 recipe
Calories per serving: 87

Sweet Potato Soup

1/2 cup chopped onion
1 tbsp vegetable oil
1 cup sliced celery (leaves and stalks)
1 lb sweet potatoes, peeled and cut into
  2-inch sections
1 1/2 cups chicken stock (homemade or
  canned)
1 bay leaf
1/2 tsp thyme
1/2 tsp rosemary
1/2 tsp ginger or mace
Salt and pepper to taste
Toasted croutons or slivers of jicama for
  garnish

1. Sauté onion in oil until golden, about 3 minutes.
2. Add all other ingredients except croutons then bring to a boil.
3. Reduce heat and simmer until potatoes are very tender. Allow to cool.
4. Remove bay leaf, then purée in batches in a processor or blender until creamy.
5. Reheat for serving. Garnish with croutons or slivers of jicama.

YIELDS: 4 SERVINGS

Nutritional breakdown: 6 grams protein, 32 grams carbohydrate, 5 grams fat
Serving portion: 1/4 recipe
Calories per serving: 192

Today's Healthy Corn Chowder

1 medium onion, diced
1/2 bell pepper, diced
2 tbsps vegetable oil
1 potato, diced
1 1/2 cups water
1 1/2 cups corn kernels, drained
1 cup chicken broth
1 tsp vegetable salt
1/4 tsp pepper, to taste

1. Sauté onion and bell pepper in oil until browned and limp.
2. Dice potato and add to water. Bring to a boil. Reduce heat and simmer until tender.
3. Place all ingredients in a blender (including potato water) and purée for approximately 15 seconds. Soup should be thick and chunky.
4. Reheat before serving.

YIELDS: 1 QUART

Nutritional breakdown: 4 grams protein, 22 grams carbohydrate, 7 grams fat
Serving: 1 cup
Calories per serving: 160

Carrot and Ginger Soup

1 medium onion, diced
4 garlic cloves, minced
2 tbsps olive oil
2 lbs carrots, cut into 1-inch chunks
2 tbsps peeled and chopped ginger root
1 qt chicken stock, defatted
Plain yogurt and sesame seeds for garnish

1. Sauté onion and garlic in oil for 5 minutes. Add carrots, cover, and cook for 15 minutes.
2. Add half the ginger and all the stock. Simmer 15 minutes.
3. Add the rest of the ginger. Purée soup in a blender or food processor.
4. Pour into bowls and garnish.

YIELDS: 6 SERVINGS

Nutritional breakdown: 5 grams protein, 18 grams carbohydrate, 6 grams fat
Serving portion: 1/6 recipe
Calories per serving: 142
Recipe courtesy Dr. Gale Shemwell-Rudolph

 # *French Bread Soup*

3 green onions
1 lb mushrooms, sliced
1 garlic clove
2 tbsps olive oil
2 tbsps tomato purée
1 tbsp sweet vermouth
2 (14 1/2-oz) cans chicken broth, defatted
4 slices French bread, toasted
1 tbsp grated Parmesan cheese

1. Lightly sauté onions, mushrooms, and garlic in hot oil.
2. Add tomato purée, vermouth, and skimmed chicken broth.
3. Simmer and serve on toasted French bread slices in soup bowls. Sprinkle with Parmesan cheese.

YIELDS: 1 QUART

Nutritional breakdown: 16 grams protein, 27 grams carbohydrate, 14 grams fat
Serving portion: 1 cup
Calories: 321
Recipe courtesy Pat Rettig

⊡ *Old-Fashioned Chicken Soup* *(with Matzo Balls)*

2 1/2 to 3 lbs chicken, cut up
1 1/2 tsps vegetable salt
1/4 tsp pepper
1/4 tsp basil (optional)
1 bay leaf
4 medium carrots
1/2 lb small white onions
1 cup fine noodles, uncooked, or matzo balls
(see following recipe)
1 tbsp finely chopped parsley

1. Wash chicken. Place in a large kettle and cover with 5 cups water. Add seasonings.
2. Simmer, covered, 1 1/2 hours, or until chicken is tender.
3. While chicken is cooking, prepare vegetables: wash and scrub carrots, cut into 1-inch chunks. Wash and peel onions.
4. When chicken is done, remove it, along with bay leaf, from stock. Skim off as much fat as possible from stock.
5. Bring back to a boil. Add carrots and onions; simmer 45 minutes.
6. While vegetables are cooking, remove skin and bones from chicken, leaving chicken in large pieces. Save scraps for sandwiches or salad.
7. Ten minutes before vegetables are done, add noodles or matzo balls and chicken pieces. Cook 10 minutes longer.
8. Sprinkle with parsley.

YIELDS: 4 SERVINGS

Nutritional breakdown: 18 grams protein, 20 grams carbohydrate, 5 grams fat
Serving portion: 1/4 recipe
Calories per serving: 203
Recipe courtesy Giselle Ganes

To flavor rice, cook in chicken broth or bouillon.

Matzo Balls

2 eggs
2 tbsps vegetable oil
I tsp salt
1/2 cup matzo meal
2 tbsps chicken broth (canned may be used)

1. Beat the eggs and add vegetable oil.
2. Mix salt with matzo meal.
3. Pour matzo meal into egg mixture and mix thoroughly. Add broth and mix once more.
4. Refrigerate at least I hour or more.
5. Form into 12 balls the size of walnuts and toss into 4 quarts salted boiling water. Cover and cook on medium flame for I hour. Drain and use in soup, especially Old-Fashioned Chicken Soup (opposite).

YIELDS: 12 MATZO BALLS

Nutritional breakdown: 5 grams protein, 12 grams carbohydrate, 10 grams fat
Serving portion: 3 matzo balls
Calories per serving: 157

Broccoli Spinach Soup

2 heads broccoli, tough ends trimmed away
I large onion, chopped
2 leeks, sliced thin
I carrot, diced
6 garlic cloves, minced
2 to 3 tbsps olive oil
8 cups chicken stock
2 plum tomatoes, chopped
1/4 cup chopped Italian parsley
I bunch (12 oz) fresh spinach, chopped
1/4 tsp nutmeg
1/4 tsp cardamom
Freshly ground pepper
1/4 cup fresh lemon juice

1. Peel broccoli stems, chop florets, and thinly slice stems. Set aside.
2. Sauté onion, leeks, carrot, and garlic in olive oil over low heat, covered, until wilted—about 10 minutes.
3. Add stock, broccoli, tomato, and parsley. Bring to a boil.
4. Simmer, covered, for 25 minutes. Wash and chop spinach and remove tough ends. Add spinach to soup. Stir in nutmeg, cardamom, pepper, and lemon juice.
5. Cook for I minute and remove from heat. Serve.

YIELDS: 8 SERVINGS

Nutritional breakdown: 7 grams protein, 13 grams carbohydrate, 6 grams fat
Serving portion: 1/8 recipe
Calories per serving: 128
Recipe courtesy Lucy Thomas, Louisiana Pacific Corp.

Open-Face Cucumber Sandwiches

1 slice whole wheat or whole grain bread
1/2 cucumber
1 tbsp light mayonnaise

1. Using a 2-inch juice glass, cut out bread circles.
2. Take a fork and score washed cucumber. Slice 1/8 inch thick and place on bread rounds.
3. Add a dollop of light mayonnaise on each and top with one or more of the following: baby shrimp, pimiento strips, caviar, carrot curl, fresh dill, alfalfa sprouts.
4. Or substitute cottage cheese, yogurt, or half yogurt and half mayonnaise, or half mayonnaise and half Dijon mustard.

YIELDS: 1 SERVING

Nutritional breakdown: 4 grams protein, 18 grams carbohydrate, 5 grams fat
Serving portion: 1 sandwich
Calories per serving: 128

 # *Tangy Pocket Burgers*

1 cup shredded cabbage
1/2 cup shredded carrots
1/4 cup sliced radishes
3 tbsps minced parsley
1 cup plain low-fat yogurt
Dash of pepper
1 lb ground beef (or turkey)
3/4 cup Quaker Oats (quick or
 old-fashioned, uncooked)
1/4 cup finely chopped onion
Dash of pepper
6 lettuce leaves
3 pita loaves, cut in half
1 large tomato, sliced

1. Combine cabbage, carrots, radishes, 1 tbsp parsley, 1/2 cup yogurt, and pepper; mix well. Chill.
2. Combine beef (or turkey), oats, remaining 1/2 cup yogurt, onion, remaining parsley, and pepper. Shape mixture into six 1/2-inch-thick patties; place on rack of broiler pan about 4 inches from heat. Broil 3 to 4 minutes on each side, or until of desired doneness.
3. Place each burger in lettuce-lined pita half; top with a tomato slice and 1/4 cup vegetable mixture.

YIELDS: 6 BURGERS

Nutritional breakdown: 26 grams protein, 24 grams carbohydrate, 14 grams fat
Serving portion: 1 burger
Calories per serving: 310
Recipe courtesy Quaker Oats Company

Crustless Chard Quiche

1 lb Swiss chard leaves or spinach
3 large eggs, or 5 egg whites
1 cup grated Parmesan cheese
2 tbsps chicken broth
Salt and pepper to taste
2 tbsps toasted pine nuts to garnish

1. Wash and chop chard. Sauté in a skillet until wilted. Set aside.
2. Combine eggs and cheese in a blender. Add chard and chicken broth. Season to taste.
3. Pour into prepared 8-inch pie pan (crust or crustless).
4. Bake at 400 degrees 25 minutes or until set.
5. Garnish with pine nuts.

YIELDS: 6 SERVINGS

Nutritional breakdown: 16 grams protein, 27 grams carbohydrate, 22 grams fat
Serving portion: 1/6 pie
Calories per serving: 351
Recipe courtesy Bob and Mary Parkhouse

Mouth-Watering Chicken Sandwich

1 whole wheat or sourdough roll
1 tbsp alfalfa sprouts
1 cup thinly sliced cooked chicken
  (approximately a 3-oz chicken breast)
1 tomato, sliced

Vinaigrette:

1/4 cup olive oil
3 tbsps red wine vinegar
2 tsps Dijon mustard

1. Brush bread or roll with 1 tablespoon vinaigrette dressing.
2. Layer sprouts, chicken, more vinaigrette, and top with sliced tomato.

YIELDS: 1 SERVING

Nutritional breakdown (without vinaigrette): 31 grams protein, 24 grams carbohydrate, 11 grams fat
Serving portion: 1 sandwich
Calories per serving: 318
Note: Each tablespoon of vinaigrette adds 7 grams fat and 63 additional calories.

⟨image⟩ *Tofu Patty*

1 (16-oz) carton tofu (drain off water)
2 green onions, chopped fine
4 eggs, or 6 egg whites
1/2 lb mushrooms, sliced
1/2 lb bean sprouts
Salt to taste
1 can water chestnuts, sliced
Optional: crabmeat or shrimp (1 can, drained)
2 tbsps safflower oil

1. Mix together all ingredients except oil.
2. Form into patties.
3. Pour safflower oil into a hot skillet. Heat patties on both sides.
4. Drain on paper towels and keep warm while frying more.
5. Serve immediately.

YIELDS: 4 SERVINGS

Nutritional breakdown: 24 grams protein, 13 grams carbohydrate, 11 grams fat
Serving portion: 1/4 recipe
Calories per serving: 237
Recipe courtesy Norma Fulvio

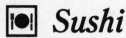 *Sushi*

1/4 cup vinegar
1/4 cup honey
2 cups cooked brown rice
1 (10-ct) pkg seaweed (nori)
5 oz fresh tuna
1 cucumber
1 avocado

1. Mix vinegar and honey together and stir into cooked rice.
2. Spread out seaweed. Spread rice mixture in a thin layer on top of seaweed.
3. Lay sushi ingredients (slice of tuna or other fresh seafood) along with a slice of cucumber or avocado on top of rice mixture.
4. Roll seaweed tightly and moisten end flap. Slice to desired thickness.
Optional:
Dip in soy sauce and/or wasabi (Japanese horseradish).

YIELDS: 5 SERVINGS

Nutritional breakdown: 6 grams protein, 35 grams carbohydrate, 1 gram fat
Serving portion: 2 rolls
Calories per serving: 168

▣ *Italian Shrimp Pizza*

There is no need to go out and buy a fancy baking tile to produce a crisp bottom on your pizza. An unglazed terra-cotta tile purchased from a flooring or tile store can work just as well.

Crust:

1 cup warm water
1 pkg active dry yeast
1 1/2 cups unbleached all-purpose flour
1 cup whole wheat flour
1 tbsp olive oil

Toppings:

1/2 cup bay shrimp
8 sun-dried tomatoes
1 chopped leek
2 garlic cloves, minced
1/4 cup chopped sweet red onion
1/2 cup sliced mushrooms (sautéed in 2 tsps olive oil)
2 tbsps chopped fresh basil

1. Combine water, yeast, and all-purpose flour in a large bowl. Mix well.
2. Add whole wheat flour and oil. Work with hands or a wooden spoon until dough holds its shape.
3. Place dough on a lightly floured surface and knead until it becomes smooth and elastic (roughly 5 minutes). If dough becomes sticky, sprinkle on a bit more flour.
4. Transfer dough to a bowl that is lightly covered with oil and let it sit, covered, in a warm place for an hour, or until it has roughly doubled in size.
5. When the dough has risen, divide it into halves. Roll each half into the shape of a pizza crust and then cover with a towel for 15 to 20 minutes.
6. Preheat oven to 500 degrees an hour in advance.
7. Transfer pizza crust to a pizza pan and brush the top of the crust with olive oil. Top with small shrimp, sun-dried tomatoes, leek, garlic, onion, sautéed mushrooms, and fresh basil.
8. Bake for 20 to 25 minutes, until golden brown.

YIELDS: 4 SERVINGS (2 PIZZAS)

Nutritional breakdown: 16 grams protein, 74 grams carbohydrate, 11 grams fat
Serving portion: 1/2 pizza
Calories per serving: 446
Recipe courtesy Lucy Thomas, Louisiana Pacific Corp.

Add lemon juice to cooking liquid when poaching fish for a firmer, whiter look.

🍽 *Spinach Manfredo*

1 garlic clove, minced
1 tbsp olive oil
Salt and pepper to taste
1 bunch fresh spinach (12 oz)

1. Brown garlic in olive oil. Add seasoning and toss in clean, wet spinach leaves.
2. Cover. Reduce heat and steam until wilted.
3. Toss again.

Note: Hot red pepper flakes add a nice bite. Add according to taste.

YIELDS: 2 SERVINGS

Nutritional breakdown: 5 grams protein, 6 grams carbohydrate, 7 grams fat
Serving portion: 1/2 recipe
Calories per serving: 100
Recipe courtesy Mary Ann Manfredo

8 Dinner, Side Dishes, and Breads

 ## *Hasty Tasty Game Hens*

1/4 cup oriental sesame oil
1/4 cup light soy sauce
2 plump Cornish game hens, each split in
  half

1. Combine oil and soy sauce to make marinade. Coat halves of hens and marinate in a 1-gallon plastic bag for 15 minutes or longer.
2. Place hens in a baking dish, cavity side down. Bake at 375 degrees for approximately 30 minutes. Turn off heat and allow birds to remain in oven for an additional 30 minutes, or until juices run clear.

YIELDS: 4 SERVINGS

Nutritional breakdown: 13 grams protein, 2 grams carbohydrate, 20 grams fat
Serving portion: 1/2 game hen
Calories per serving: 242

Danny's Roasted Chicken

Garlic powder
Teriyaki sauce
1 3- to 3 1/2-lb whole chicken

1. Mix garlic powder with teriyaki sauce and brush on chicken.
2. Place chicken in a foil tent. Bake about 1 hour at 450 degrees. For the final 15 minutes, open foil and allow chicken to brown.

Hint:

To lower fat content of chicken, bake the bird on a vertical roasting rack. This allows the fat to drain from the chicken as it bakes.

YIELDS: 4 SERVINGS

Nutritional breakdown: with skin, 46 grams protein, 0 grams carbohydrate, 16 grams fat; without skin, 46 grams protein, 0 grams carbohydrate, 10 grams fat
Serving portion: 1/4 chicken
Calories per serving: with skin, 380; without skin, 288
Recipe courtesy Dan Doyle

For moist chicken, cook with the skin on. Remove the skin before serving.

Jack's Chop-Chop with Spaghetti and Chicken

Use any or all of the following vegetables; chop the vegetables bite-size and gauge the volume on how many people you wish to serve (1 1/2 cups raw vegetables and 1 cup cooked pasta equals 2 servings):

Carrots, cauliflower, bean sprouts, mushrooms, broccoli, turnips, green onions or leeks, jicama, bell peppers (green or red), celery, red cabbage, swiss chard, goose-neck squash, pea pods, baby asparagus, zucchini

2 half chicken breasts minus skin, cut into bite-size pieces
Soy sauce
Wine
Garlic powder (optional)
Chopped parsley (optional)
2 to 3 tbsps safflower oil
1 cup cooked pasta

1. Marinate chicken in soy sauce and wine to taste. You can season with garlic powder and parsley.
2. Put 2 to 3 tablespoons safflower oil in a wok or skillet.
3. Using high heat, sauté all the vegetables (except bean sprouts and mushrooms, which should go in late in the sautéing process).
4. Sauté until vegetables are crispy and heated throughout. Add chicken. Stir constantly.
5. Serve over wheat/soy spaghetti.

YIELDS: 2 SERVINGS

Nutritional breakdown: 14 grams protein, 24 grams carbohydrate, 12 grams fat
Serving portion: 1/2 recipe
Calories per serving: 314

Chicken Adobo

1 chicken, approximately 3 lbs, skinned and cut up
1/4 cup soy sauce (for color)
2 tbsps vinegar
1/4 tsp ground pepper
3 bay leaves
3 crushed garlic cloves
1/3 cup water
2 cups cooked brown rice

1. Place all ingredients (except rice) into a pot and boil, covered, for 30 minutes.
2. Reduce to a simmer and continue cooking for 30 additional minutes.
3. Serve over the rice.

YIELDS: 4 SERVINGS

Nutritional breakdown: 16 grams protein, 34 grams carbohydrate, 3 grams fat
Serving portion: 1/4 recipe
Calories per serving: 231
Recipe courtesy Terry Ganes

◉ Raechel's Tamale Pie

1 whole chicken
3 large onions
Salt and pepper (optional)
2 garlic cloves
1 1/2 cups sliced fresh mushrooms
1 cup light olive oil
1 large (32-oz) can tomato purée (or 4 cups homemade purée)
3 level tbsps chili powder
2 cups yellow cornmeal
Optional: 1 small package frozen corn; 1 can sliced olives

1. In a large covered pot, boil whole chicken, 1 chopped onion, salt, and pepper to taste in water, until tender. Allow to stand in broth until cool. Remove chicken from broth, remove skin, debone, and shred.
2. Chill broth in refrigerator until fat rises to surface.
3. Sauté 2 chopped onions, garlic, and mushrooms in olive oil until tender. Set aside.
4. Bring tomato purée, chili powder, salt, and pepper to a boil. Reduce heat. Simmer 15 minutes, stirring frequently. Set aside.
5. Skim fat from chilled broth (you should have about 1 quart) and bring broth to a boil. Slowly pour in the cornmeal, stirring constantly, until bubbles break. Remove from heat.
6. Mix all prepared ingredients together. Pour into a 9 x 13-inch baking dish.
7. Bake in a 350-degree oven until dish is hot throughout.

YIELDS: 12 SERVINGS

Nutritional breakdown: 20 grams protein, 16 grams carbohydrate, 22 grams fat
Serving portion: 1/12 recipe
Calories per serving: 328
Recipe courtesy Raechel Parker

Luscious Lemon Chicken

2 whole boned chicken breasts, cut into 4
 pieces
1/2 cup lemon juice
1 tsp dill weed
1 tsp thyme
1 tsp basil
1/4 tsp oregano
1/4 tsp garlic powder
Salt (optional)

1. Lightly coat a 1- or 1 1/2-quart square baking dish with vegetable oil. Fit in the chicken breasts so they are compact.
2. Pour on lemon juice. Sprinkle with herbs. Marinate in the refrigerator overnight.
3. Bake in a preheated 375-degree oven for 20 to 30 minutes.

YIELDS: 4 SERVINGS

Nutritional breakdown: 27 grams protein, 3 grams carbohydrate, 3 grams fat
Serving portion: 1/4 recipe
Calories per serving: 153

 # *Golden Glazed Chicken*

6 chicken legs with thighs
1/4 cup slivered almonds

Mustard sauce:

1/2 cup honey
1/2 cup Dijon mustard
1 tsp lemon juice
1 tsp finely chopped onion
1/2 tsp curry powder, or to taste

1. Place legs with thighs in a baking dish lightly coated with vegetable oil. Combine mustard sauce ingredients and spoon over chicken.
2. Bake in a preheated 400-degree oven for 30 minutes. Baste periodically.
3. Sprinkle with slivered almonds and return to oven for another 10 minutes with heat turned off.
Note: To reduce fat content and lower calories, remove chicken skin and delete almonds.

YIELDS: 6 SERVINGS

Nutritional breakdown: 32 grams protein, 25 grams carbohydrate, 19 grams fat
Serving portion: 1/6 recipe
Calories per serving: 400

◙ *Chicken Oriental*

1/2 cup chopped celery
1/2 tsp chopped fresh ginger, or 1/4 tsp
    ground ginger
1 garlic clove, finely chopped
2 tbsps olive oil
4 skinless, boneless chicken breast halves,
    cut into bite-size pieces
1 large green or red bell pepper, cut into
    slices
1/2 cup chopped green onion
1/2 cup sliced water chestnuts
1/4 lb snow peas, cleaned and strings
    removed
1/2 cup diced jicama (optional)
2 tbsps oriental sesame oil
1 tbsp light soy sauce

1. Sauté celery, ginger, and garlic in olive oil.
2. Add chicken, peppers, green onion, water chestnuts, snow peas (and jicama if desired). Stir-fry until chicken is cooked and vegetables are tender but still crisp.
3. Just before serving, combine sesame oil and soy sauce and pour over chicken and vegetables. Stir and serve.

YIELDS: 6 SERVINGS

Nutritional breakdown: 37 grams protein, 6 grams carbohydrate, 13 grams fat
Serving portion: 1/6 recipe
Calories per serving: 297

◙ *Chicken Curry*

1 medium onion, sliced
Vegetable oil
6 to 8 chicken pieces
1 green bell pepper, seeded and chopped
1 apple, diced
1/2 cup chopped celery
1 tbsp curry powder

1. Sauté onion in a small amount of vegetable oil until tender.
2. Add chicken pieces and brown.
3. Add chopped bell pepper, apple, celery, and curry powder. Cover and cook until chicken is tender. More water may be added if desired.
4. Serve with rice and raw vegetable salad.

YIELDS: 3 TO 4 SERVINGS

Nutritional breakdown: 31 grams protein, 7 grams carbohydrate, 7 grams fat
Serving portion: 2 chicken pieces
Calories per serving: 220

Mexicali Chicken Breasts

1/2 cup Quaker Oats (quick or
 old-fashioned, uncooked)
1 tbsp minced parsley
3/4 tsp chili powder
3/4 tsp paprika
2 chicken breasts, split and skinned
3 tbsps margarine, melted
2 medium tomatoes, coarsely chopped
1/2 cup chopped green bell pepper
1/4 cup coarsely chopped onion
2 tbsps minced parsley
1 small garlic clove, minced
1 tbsp lemon juice

1. Heat oven to 425 degrees.
2. Place oats, parsley, and seasoning in a blender or food processor; blend about 1 minute, stopping occasionally to stir. Coat chicken with oat mixture. Place on a rack in a 15 x 10-inch jelly roll pan; gently brush entire surface of chicken with margarine.
3. Bake 35 to 40 minutes, or until juices run clear when chicken is pierced with a fork.
4. Meanwhile, combine remaining ingredients; mix well. Serve with chicken.

YIELDS: 4 SERVINGS

Nutritional breakdown: 29 grams protein, 10 grams carbohydrate, 12 grams fat
Serving portion: 1/2 chicken breast and garnish
Calories per serving: 270
Recipe courtesy Quaker Oats Company

Eric's Tantalizing Turkey Loaf

1 1/2 lbs ground turkey (or lean beef)
1 cup fine bulgur
1 (15-oz) can tomato sauce
2 egg whites
1 onion, finely chopped
1 garlic clove (optional)
1/2 tsp thyme
1/2 tsp rosemary
1/2 tsp oregano
1/2 tsp pepper
1 tsp vegetable salt
1/4 bell pepper, grated (red or green)
1/4 cup chopped parsley

1. Spray a standard loaf pan with cooking spray.
2. Combine all ingredients in a bowl; mix well.
3. Spoon into loaf pan and bake at 350 degrees for approximately 1 hour.
4. Drain any excess liquid and invert on a serving platter. Garnish with fresh parsley.

YIELDS: 8 SERVINGS

Nutritional breakdown: 29 grams protein, 16 grams carbohydrate, 5 grams fat
Serving portions: 1/8 loaf
Calories per serving: 223
Recipe courtesy Eric Garlick

▣ Turkey Cranberry Cutlets

1 medium orange, cut in half
1 cup fresh or frozen cranberries
1 tsp grated orange peel
1/4 cup sugar
1 cup Quaker Oats (quick or old-fashioned, uncooked)
1 tbsp minced parsley
1/2 tsp poultry seasoning
1 lb fresh turkey breast slices
3 tbsps vegetable oil

1. Juice half the orange; set aside.
2. Scoop out pulp from remaining orange half.
3. Place cranberries, orange pulp, grated orange peel, and sugar in a blender or food processor. Blend on medium speed about 30 seconds, or until mixture is coarsely chopped.
4. Combine oats and seasonings in a blender or food processor; cover. Blend about 1 minute, stopping occasionally to stir.
5. Dip each turkey slice in reserved orange juice; coat with oat mixture. Sauté in oil over medium heat 2 to 3 minutes on each side, or until evenly browned and tender. Serve with sauce.

YIELDS: 4 SERVINGS

Nutritional breakdown: 39 grams protein, 31 grams carbohydrate, 13 grams fat
Serving portion: 2 turkey slices, 1/4 cup sauce
Calories per serving: 380
Recipe courtesy Quaker Oats Company

Fresh Sauce

Fresh Sauce has multiple uses—as a topping for Eric's Tantalizing Turkey Loaf, eggplant, tofu, or pasta.

1/2 garlic clove, minced
1 green onion
2 fresh medium tomatoes
4 to 6 fresh basil leaves
1/2 bunch parsley
1/2 cup vegetable bouillon or chicken broth

Coarsely chop onion, tomatoes, basil, and parsley. Sauté with garlic in bouillon until tender-crisp.

Variation:

Include additional vegetables or clams.

YIELDS: 2 CUPS

Nutritional breakdown: 3 grams protein, 14 grams carbohydrate, 0 grams fat
Serving portion: 1 tablespoon
Calories per serving: 70
Recipe courtesy Susan LaLanne

◉ *Spaghetti Sauce for an Army*

5 tbsps olive oil
1 onion, chopped
2 tbsps minced garlic
2 lbs ground turkey (or lean ground beef)
3 (28-oz) cans tomato sauce
3 (12-oz) cans tomato paste
1 (28-oz) can crushed tomatoes
3 tbsps Italian seasoning
2 to 3 dozen aniseeds
1 tbsp oregano
1 tbsp thyme
1 tsp rosemary

1. Pour olive oil into a very large pot over low heat. Sauté onion and garlic until lightly browned.
2. In a skillet, sauté ground turkey (or beef), pouring off excess liquid. Set aside.
3. Pour cans of tomato sauce, tomato paste, and crushed tomatoes into the pot with olive oil, onion, and garlic, continuing with low heat. Add all seasonings. Add turkey.
4. Simmer for 2 hours, stirring periodically to mix ingredients and to prevent sticking.

YIELDS: 5 QUARTS

Nutritional breakdown: 9 grams protein, 12 grams carbohydrate, 4 grams fat
Serving portion: 1/2 cup
Calories per serving: 111
Recipe courtesy Richard Benyo

To make peeling tomatoes easier, briefly submerge them in boiling water, then immediately dip them into cold water. This hot/cold treatment cracks the skin and greatly speeds the peeling process.

Elaine's Stuffed Cabbage

Sauce:

1 (16-oz) can tomato sauce
1 1/2 cups water
2/3 cup honey
3/4 cup cider vinegar

1 large cabbage (or 1 1/2 lbs cabbage leaves)
3/4 to 1 lb ground turkey
1 or 2 egg whites
1 onion, chopped
1 cup grated carrots
1 cup cooked brown rice, or 1 cup cooked
 wheat berries (whole grain wheat)
Salt and pepper to taste
1/4 tsp cloves (optional)
1/4 cup chopped nuts (optional)

1. To make sauce, combine ingredients and bring to a boil. Reduce heat and simmer for 10 minutes.
2. Bring 2 quarts water to a boil. Remove cabbage leaves from head. Cut leaves off as you peel them so as not to break the leaves. Wash and blanch in boiling water until manageable. Drain leaves, set aside.
3. Combine filling ingredients, mixing well.
4. Place 2 heaping tablespoons meat mixture on each leaf. Roll, folding ends or rolls over, and fasten with toothpicks. Place seam down in a baking dish. Pour sauce over rolls.
5. Cover and bake at 350 degrees for 30 minutes.
6. Uncover and cook for 10 additional minutes.

YIELDS: 4 SERVINGS

Nutritional breakdown: 31 grams protein, 40 grams carbohydrate, 7 grams fat
Serving portion: 1/4 recipe
Calories per serving: 326

Surprise Meatballs

12 plump California prunes
1 slice fresh pineapple
1 egg
1 1/2 lbs ground beef or ground turkey
1/2 cup fine dry bread crumbs
1/4 to 1/2 cup skim milk
1 1/2 tsps vegetable salt
Dash of pepper
1 tbsp cooking oil (olive, soy, or safflower)
1/2 cup sliced fresh mushrooms
1 cup water
1 tbsp whole grain flour
Arrowroot (optional)

1. Pit prunes and stuff each with a small wedge (approximately 1 tablespoon) of pineapple.
2. Beat egg lightly and blend with ground beef or turkey, crumbs, milk, salt, and pepper. Shape mixture around stuffed prunes into balls, covering prune completely.
3. Sauté on all sides in a small amount of hot oil.
4. Add mushrooms and water, cover closely, and cook slowly for 20 to 30 minutes.
5. Option: thicken sauce with arrowroot mixed with water.

YIELDS: 6 SERVINGS

Nutritional breakdown: 38 grams protein, 22 grams carbohydrate, 14 grams fat
Serving portion: 2 meatballs
Calories per serving: 364

Wheat Chili

2 to 2 1/2 lbs ground turkey or hamburger
1 to 2 medium onions
1 green bell pepper, chopped
1 fresh tomato, chopped
1 1/2 tsps salt
1/4 tsp pepper
2 tsps chili powder (or to taste)
2 garlic cloves, minced (or 1/2 tsp granulated garlic)
1 (15-oz) can tomato sauce
1 (15-oz) can chicken broth
1 cup tomato paste
3 cups cooked whole wheat berries (whole grain wheat)

1. Brown turkey or hamburger (if turkey, add a small amount of water or chicken broth to prevent sticking).
2. Add remaining ingredients and simmer for 45 minutes to blend flavors.

YIELDS: 24 SERVINGS

Nutritional breakdown: 40 grams protein, 29 grams carbohydrate, 7 grams fat
Serving portion: 1/2 cup
Calories per serving: 334

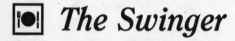 Turkey Soup

This recipe is here instead of in chapter 7 with the other soups because when Jack and I make this turkey soup, we use it as a main course. Just add some nutritious bread and you've got a whole meal.

Turkey carcass
2 onions, chopped
1 tsp salt
Pinch of rosemary, basil, garlic powder to
  taste
1 bay leaf
1 cup cut carrots
1 cup cubed squash
1 cup cut broccoli
1 cup cut napa cabbage
6 cups any additional cut up vegetable
  (jicama, bell pepper, celery, zucchini,
  potato, turnip, mushrooms, etc.)

1. Boil turkey carcass in water to cover with 1 chopped onion and salt until the meat falls off the bone. Discard the bones and season the broth to taste with rosemary, basil, garlic powder; add bay leaf.
2. Cool and skim off any excess fat from broth.
3. Add remaining chopped onion and the carrots, squash, broccoli, and napa cabbage. Reheat.
4. Add 6 cups of additional vegetables of your choice. Simmer until vegetables are tender. Add additional seasoning to taste.

YIELDS: 3 QUARTS

Nutritional breakdown: 5 grams protein, 9 grams carbohydrate, 1 gram fat
Serving portion: 1 cup
Calories per serving: 58

◙ The Swinger

1/3 to 1/2 lb ground beef or turkey
1 egg
1/2 cup total of mix of the following: diced
  green bell pepper, Cheddar cheese
  (grated), chopped onion, chopped tomato,
  sliced olives
Pinch of sea salt to taste
2 tsps wheat germ
2 whole wheat rolls, or 2 pieces toasted
  whole wheat bread (optional)
Alfalfa sprouts to garnish

1. Place all ingredients except rolls or bread into a mixing bowl and mix together well.
2. Form into 2 patties and broil to preferred doneness.
3. Serve as you would a hamburger, or serve open-faced on toasted whole wheat bread. Garnish with alfalfa sprouts.

YIELDS: 2 SERVINGS

Nutritional breakdown: 40 grams protein, 16 grams carbohydrate, 32 grams fat
Serving portion: 1 burger
Calories per serving: 514
Recipe courtesy Jim Baker

Veal Stew

3 tbsps corn oil
2 lbs boneless veal, cut into 1-inch cubes
1 1/2 cups chopped onion
1/4 tsp pepper
1 1/2 cups chicken bouillon or vegetable
 broth
1/2 cup white wine
1/2 lb celery, cut into 1-inch slices
1/2 tsp dried dill weed
1/2 lb mushrooms, cut in half
1 (10-oz) pkg frozen peas, thawed

1. Heat corn oil in a Dutch oven over medium heat. Add veal. Brown well. Pour off excess fat.
2. Stir in chopped onion and pepper. Add bouillon and wine. Cover.
3. Bake in a 350-degree oven for 45 minutes.
4. Add celery. Cover and cook 20 to 30 minutes longer, or until meat and vegetables are tender.
5. Add remaining ingredients. Cover. Cook 5 to 10 minutes, or until vegetables are tender.
6. Make the dish ahead of time, chill it, then remove any congealed fat before reheating.

YIELDS: 6 SERVINGS

Nutritional breakdown: 25 grams protein, 13 grams carbohydrate, 15 grams fat
Serving portion: 1/6 recipe
Calories per serving: 320
Recipe courtesy Mazola corn oil

Steak and Veggies

1 1/2 lbs sirloin steak (trimmed)
3 tbsps safflower oil
1/8 tsp vegetable salt
1/8 tsp pepper
2 cups diagonally sliced celery
1 medium green bell pepper, cut into
 1/4-inch strips (2 cups)
1 cup finely chopped green onions
1 garlic clove, minced

1. Cut meat into 2 1/4-inch strips.
2. In a large skillet, heat oil over medium-high heat. Add meat and cook, stirring constantly, until browned. Sprinkle with salt and pepper to taste, add celery, green pepper, green onions, and garlic, stirring constantly until vegetables are barely tender.

Variation:
————
Add sliced fresh mushrooms, bamboo shoots, sliced fresh bean sprouts, or water chestnuts.

YIELDS: 6 SERVINGS

Nutritional breakdown: 35 grams protein, 4 grams carbohydrate, 21 grams fat
Serving portion: 1/6 recipe
Calories per serving: 347

Roast Stuffed Leg of Lamb with Broiled Tomatoes

6 1/2 oz cubed whole wheat toast or whole wheat stuffing mix
1/2 tsp crushed rosemary
1/2 cup sliced celery
1/2 cup chopped onion
1/2 cup chopped green bell pepper
1/4 cup cooking oil (canola, olive, or safflower)
2 egg whites
1/2 to 3/4 cup tomato juice
1 (6-lb) leg of lamb, boned and fat trimmed
6 fresh tomatoes

1. Put bread cubes into a bowl. Add crushed rosemary, celery, onion, and green pepper. Stir in oil, egg whites, and tomato juice. Mix thoroughly.
2. Fill lamb pocket (where bone was) with filling. Tie or fasten with skewers.
3. Shape remaining dressing into rounds and place in a covered baking dish.
4. Place lamb on a rack, fat side up, in an open roasting pan. Roast at 325 degrees for about 3 hours, or until meat thermometer reads 182 degrees.
5. During last 30 minutes of roasting time, bake dressing rounds and serve on broiled tomato halves.

Hint:

For a more colorful meal, serve with steamed seasoned Brussels sprouts.

YIELDS: 12 SERVINGS

Nutritional breakdown: 35 grams protein, 12 grams carbohydrate, 16 grams fat
Serving portion: 1/12 recipe
Calories per serving: 336

Use bran in meatloaf, meatballs, etc., as a hardy, tasty way to guarantee your daily fiber requirements.

Andy's Broiled Lamb Chops

4 spring lamb chops, cut from the leg (3/4 inch thick)
4 tsps prepared mustard
4 tsps cider vinegar
4 tsps honey
Vegetable salt to taste (optional)

1. Trim excess fat from chops; slash edges of chops in several places to prevent curling.
2. In a small bowl, combine mustard, vinegar, and honey for glaze.
3. Preheat broiler. Broil chops 4 inches from heat source for 5 minutes. Brush chops with half of glaze; sprinkle with salt. Broil 3 minutes longer. Turn chops. Broil 4 minutes. Brush with remaining glaze, sprinkle with vegetable salt, if desired, and broil 2 minutes longer, or until chops are slightly pink in center.

Variation:

Substitute 4 teaspoons horseradish for vinegar and honey.

YIELDS: 2 SERVINGS

Nutritional breakdown: 32 grams protein, 12 grams carbohydrate, 15 grams fat
Serving portion: 2 chops
Calories per serving: 321
Recipe courtesy Andy Rorem

Fish Fillets Italiano

1 1/4 cups Quaker Oats (quick or
  old-fashioned, uncooked)
2 tbsps grated Parmesan cheese
1 tsp Italian seasoning
1/8 tsp garlic powder
2 tbsps margarine
2 small zucchini, cut into 1/4-inch strips
6 sole or flounder fillets (about 1 1/4 lbs)
2 tbsps lemon juice

1. Sauté oats, cheese, and seasonings in margarine, stirring frequently until golden brown; set aside.
2. Heat oven to 375 degrees. Sprinkle zucchini evenly over fish fillets. Roll up, beginning at wide end; secure with toothpicks. Place seam side down in an 8- or 9-inch glass baking dish; sprinkle with lemon juice. Cover with aluminum foil.
3. Bake 20 to 25 minutes, until fish fillets turn opaque; remove to a serving plate. Top with oat mixture. Serve with lemon wedges, if desired.

YIELDS: 6 SERVINGS

Nutritional breakdown: 28 grams protein, 12 grams carbohydrate, 7 grams fat
Serving portion: 1 stuffed sole fillet
Calories per serving: 210
Recipe courtesy Quaker Oats Company

Mollie's Classic Poached Salmon

1 quart water
1 cup white wine
4 bay leaves
3 tbsps chopped parsley
4 whole peppercorns
1 tsp salt (if desired)
4 (1 inch thick) salmon steaks
  (approximately 2 lbs)
Juice of 1 lemon
1 tbsp canola oil

1. In a deep skillet, bring water, wine, bay leaves, 2 tablespoons of the chopped parsley, peppercorns, and salt to a boil.
2. Add salmon, cover, reduce heat to poach for approximately 10 minutes for each 1 inch thickness of fish.
3. Remove salmon to a platter.
4. Reserve 1/2 cup poaching liquid in skillet. Add the lemon juice and canola oil. Whisk together and add remaining 1 tablespoon parsley. Pour sauce over salmon or serve separately.

YIELDS: 4 SERVINGS

Nutritional breakdown: 38 grams protein, 1 gram carbohydrate, 23 grams fat
Serving portion: 1 salmon steak
Calories per serving: 413
Recipe courtesy Mollie Qvale

Broiled or Barbecued White Fish

1/2 cup olive oil
1/2 cup soy sauce
1/4 tsp pepper
1/4 tsp garlic powder
1 lb solid white fish (albacore, halibut, tuna, swordfish, mahi-mahi)

1. Mix olive oil, soy sauce, pepper, and garlic powder. Pour over fish and allow to marinate in refrigerator for 2 hours.
2. Fish may be baked, broiled, or barbecued.

YIELDS: 4 SERVINGS

Nutritional breakdown: 24 grams protein, 3 grams carbohydrate, 27 grams fat
Serving portion: 1/4 recipe
Calories per serving: 351
Recipe courtesy Phyllis Dorn

 # Scampi

1 1/2 lbs medium shrimp
1/2 cup olive oil
8 shallots, chopped very fine (about 3/4 cup)
4 garlic cloves, chopped fine
1 cup canned stewed tomatoes
1/2 cup sliced mushrooms
1 tsp salt
Dash of pepper
1/3 cup lemon juice
1/4 cup chopped parsley

1. Shell and devein shrimp. To butterfly, split each shrimp lengthwise, from head to tail, leaving tail intact.
2. In hot oil in a large skillet, sauté shallots and garlic, stirring, 3 minutes. Add tomatoes and mushrooms and cook, stirring, 5 minutes longer.
3. Add salt, pepper, lemon juice, 2 tablespoons of the parsley, and the shrimp. Toss to mix well.
4. Divide shrimp mixture into 6 individual baking dishes.
5. Broil, 4 to 5 inches from heat, 10 minutes, or until shrimp are tender. Sprinkle each with the rest of the parsley.

YIELDS: 6 SERVINGS

Nutritional breakdown: 23 grams protein, 9 grams carbohydrate, 19 grams fat
Serving portion: 1/6 recipe
Calories per serving: 293
Recipe courtesy Tiko Martin

California Cioppino

1/4 cup olive oil
1 celery rib, chopped
1 onion, chopped
1 garlic clove, crushed
1 leek, sliced
1 tbsp thyme
1/2 bay leaf
2 cups crushed tomatoes
1 cup clam juice
1 cup white wine
2 pinches of saffron
2 tsps chopped parsley
1/2 lb halibut chunks
1/2 lb cod chunks
1/2 lb shrimp (uncooked, peeled)
1 dozen small clams
1/2 lb scallops, quartered (optional)

1. Heat oil in a skillet and sauté celery, onion, garlic, and leek.
2. Pour the sauté mix into a large soup kettle and add everything else except seafood.
3. Simmer for 20 minutes, then add seafood.
4. Continue to simmer until all clams open. Discard any that do not open in 15 minutes. Serve in large soup bowls. This is a hearty main course served with French bread.

YIELDS: 4 SERVINGS

Nutritional breakdown: 41 grams protein, 16 grams carbohydrate, 16 grams fat
Serving portion: 1/4 recipe
Calories per serving: 402

Paella

1/4 cup unbleached flour
Salt and pepper
1 (2 1/2- to 3-pound) broiler-fryer chicken, cut up, or use 6 chicken breast halves
2 tbsps olive oil or vegetable cooking oil
2 1/2 cups chicken broth
2 medium onions, quartered
2 carrots, sliced (3/4 cup)
2/3 cup uncooked brown rice
1/2 cup chopped celery with leaves
1/4 cup chopped pimiento
1 garlic clove, minced
1/2 tsp oregano, crushed
1/4 tsp ground saffron
12 oz fresh or frozen shelled shrimp
12 small fresh clams in shells, washed
1 (9-oz) pkg frozen artichoke hearts

1. Combine flour, 1 teaspoon salt, and a dash of pepper in a paper sack. Add chicken pieces, a few at a time, shaking to coat.
2. In a 4-quart Dutch oven, brown chicken in hot oil about 15 minutes. Drain off fat.
3. Add broth, onions, carrots, rice, celery, pimiento, garlic, oregano, saffron, and 1/2 teaspoon salt. Cover; simmer 30 minutes.
4. Add shrimp, clams, and artichoke hearts.
5. Simmer, covered, 15 to 20 minutes until all clams open. Discard any that do not open.

YIELDS: 8 SERVINGS

Nutritional breakdown: 54 grams protein, 23 grams carbohydrate, 10 grams fat
Serving portion: 1/8 recipe
Calories per serving: 401
Recipe courtesy Terry Ganes

Off-the-Shelf Pasta

10 oz any pasta
2 tbsps finely chopped garlic
2 tbsps olive oil
4 cups chopped tomatoes
14 oz albacore tuna packed in water (1 large or 2 small cans)
1 to 1 1/2 cups green peas (fresh or frozen)
2 oz pimiento
2 tsps sweet dried basil

1. Cook pasta until al dente; drain and keep warm.
2. Sauté garlic in oil until translucent.
3. Add tomatoes, tuna, peas, pimiento, and basil. Cook 1 to 2 minutes.
4. Combine pasta and tuna mixture. Serve immediately.

YIELDS: 6 SERVINGS

Nutritional breakdown: 29 grams protein, 53 grams carbohydrate, 6 grams fat
Serving portion: 1/6 recipe
Calories per serving: 377

 # *Scallops Marinade*

2 lbs scallops
Juice of 2 lemons
4 garlic cloves, finely chopped

1. Marinate scallops in lemon juice and garlic for at least 1 hour.
2. Place scallops on a foil-covered baking sheet and broil for about 3 minutes, or until they turn solid white.
3. Season to taste and serve on a bed of watercress.

Variation:

Sprinkle with minced fresh parsley and slivered almonds.

YIELDS: 6 SERVINGS

Nutritional breakdown: 26 grams protein, 6 grams carbohydrate, 1 gram fat
Serving portion: 1/6 recipe
Calories per serving: 142

🍽 Fish in Foil

4 whitefish fillets (approximately 1 lb)
3 tbsps vegetable cooking oil
Freshly ground pepper
2 tbsps grated onion
2 tbsps minced parsley
4 tbsps dry white wine

1. Cut aluminum foil into four squares and fold ends over to make the shape of a boat.
2. Brush the fish with oil and place in the foil. Season each piece of fish with pepper, onion, parsley, and wine.
3. Fold over, envelope style, and be sure ends are sealed. Place on a cookie sheet and bake for 25 minutes at 425 degrees.

YIELDS: 4 SERVINGS

Nutritional breakdown: 23 grams protein, 1 gram carbohydrate, 15 grams fat
Serving portion: 1 fish fillet
Calories per serving: 244
Recipe courtesy Norma Fulvio

Rather than completely thawing frozen fish fillets, cook them when partially thawed in order to retain the essential nutrients and fluids.

Vegetable Lasagne

9 lasagne noodles (about 8 oz)
1/4 cup corn oil
3 medium onions, coarsely chopped
4 garlic cloves, minced
3 green bell peppers, coarsely chopped
3 tbsps cornstarch
1 (13 3/4- or 14 1/2-oz) can chicken broth
1 3/4 cups skim milk
1 (15-oz) container part-skim ricotta cheese
1 (10-oz) pkg frozen chopped spinach,
 thawed and well drained
3 tbsps chopped fresh basil
3/4 tsp salt
1/2 tsp nutmeg
1/2 tsp pepper
1 cup shredded part-skim mozzarella cheese

1. Cook lasagne noodles according to package directions; rinse with cold water and drain.
2. In a 6-quart Dutch oven, heat 2 tablespoons of the corn oil over medium heat. Add onions and garlic. Sauté 10 minutes, or until golden; remove.
3. Heat remaining oil in Dutch oven. Add peppers and sauté 5 minutes.
4. In a bowl, mix cornstarch and chicken broth until smooth; stir into peppers. Add milk. Stirring constantly, bring to a boil over medium heat and boil 1 minute. Remove from heat and add onions.
5. In a bowl, combine ricotta, spinach, basil, salt, nutmeg, and pepper.
6. Spoon 1 1/2 cups sauce into a 9 x 13 x 2-inch baking dish. Top with a third of the noodles and half of the spinach mixture. Repeat, beginning with sauce. Then top with remaining noodles and sauce. Sprinkle mozzarella over top.
7. Bake in a 350-degree oven 20 to 25 minutes, or until heated.

YIELDS: 10 SERVINGS

Nutritional breakdown: 16 grams protein, 28 grams carbohydrate, 13 grams fat
Serving portion: 1/10 recipe
Calories per serving: 280
Recipe courtesy Mazola corn oil

Meatless Chili

2 tbsps corn oil
1 1/2 cups chopped onions
3 garlic cloves, minced
2 tbsps chili powder
1/2 tsp ground cumin
1 cup diced carrots
1 green bell pepper, chopped
2 (14 1/2- to 16-oz) cans tomatoes in juice, undrained
1 (16-oz) can chick-peas, drained
1 (15-oz) can kidney beans, drained
1 (10-oz) pkg frozen corn, thawed
1 to 2 pickled jalapeño peppers, chopped

1. In a 5-quart saucepot, heat corn oil over medium heat. Add onions, garlic, chili powder, and cumin; sauté 5 minutes, or until tender. Add carrots and green pepper; sauté 2 minutes. Add tomatoes with juice, crushing tomatoes with a spoon. Stir in chick-peas, kidney beans, corn, and jalapeño peppers. Bring to a boil.
2. Reduce heat; cover and simmer 30 to 35 minutes. If desired, serve with rice.

YIELDS: 3 QUARTS

Nutritional breakdown: 8 grams protein, 38 grams carbohydrate, 5 grams fat
Serving portion: 1 1/2 cups
Calories per serving: 260
Recipe courtesy Mazola corn oil

Tofu Rounds in Sauce

2 tbsps oil
1 lb tofu, mashed well
2 eggs, lightly beaten
1/2 cup wheat germ
1 tsp soy sauce
1/2 tsp vegetable salt
1/4 tsp oregano
1/4 tsp basil
1/2 tsp garlic powder
3 tbsps grated Parmesan cheese
1 tbsp dehydrated onion flakes
1/4 tsp pepper
2 cups Spaghetti Sauce for an Army (page 103)

1. Combine all ingredients except spaghetti sauce in a mixing bowl.
2. Form mixture into balls about 1 inch thick.
3. Heat oil in a saucepan and brown tofu balls in hot oil.
4. Cover with sauce and serve.

YIELDS: 8 SERVINGS

Nutritional breakdown: 14 grams protein, 12 grams carbohydrate, 10 grams fat
Serving portion: 1/8 recipe
Calories per serving: 350

Italian Roll-Ups

Sauce:

1/4 cup chopped parsley
1/4 tsp salt
1 tsp dried oregano, crumbled
2 garlic cloves, chopped fine
1 bay leaf
2 tbsps finely chopped fresh basil, or 1 tsp dried
4 large ripe tomatoes, peeled, seeded, and coarsely chopped, or a 30-oz can tomato purée
Freshly ground pepper to taste

1/2 lb lasagne noodles
1/2 cup chopped onion
2 tbsps light olive oil
15 oz ricotta cheese (low-fat) and 2 egg whites, blended together
4 oz mozzarella cheese (part-skim)
1 cup thinly sliced mushrooms
1 small pkg frozen chopped spinach, thawed and drained
1/4 cup finely chopped fresh basil, or 2 tsps dried
1 1/2 tsps dried oregano, crumbled
1/4 cup finely chopped parsley
Freshly ground pepper to taste
1/4 cup grated Parmesan cheese

1. Combine all the sauce ingredients except pepper in a medium saucepan. Bring to a boil, reduce heat, and simmer for 15 minutes, stirring occasionally. Season with pepper. Set the sauce aside.
2. Preheat oven to 350 degrees.
3. Bring a large pot of water to a boil and add the noodles. Cook for 12 to 15 minutes, until noodles are tender. Drain and pat dry.
4. For filling, sauté onion in olive oil. Combine the ricotta mixture and mozzarella cheese, vegetables, herbs, and pepper in a bowl. Add sautéed onions and mix. Spoon about 1/3 cup of the mixture onto each lasagne strip, spread it over the noodle, and roll it up jelly-roll style. Spread a small amount of the sauce on the bottom of the baking dish and place the rolls in dish, seam side down. Pour remaining sauce over roll-ups and sprinkle with Parmesan cheese.
5. Bake 25 minutes, covered. Remove cover, and bake 10 to 15 minutes more, or until bubbly.

YIELDS: 12 SERVINGS

Nutritional breakdown: 10 grams protein, 11 grams carbohydrate, 8 grams fat
Serving portion: 1/12 recipe
Calories per serving: 150
Recipe courtesy Brenda Rodriques

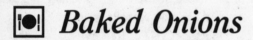 Stuffed Mushrooms

12 oz large mushrooms
1 cup whole wheat bread crumbs
2 medium tomatoes, puréed, or 1 cup
  tomato juice
1/4 cup pine nuts (or walnuts can be used)
2 tbsps chopped parsley
1/4 tsp rosemary
1 tbsp olive oil
Vegetable salt

1. Remove mushroom stems and save.
2. Wash and dry caps.
3. Chop stems and blend with remaining ingredients except vegetable salt.
4. Stuff mushrooms and sprinkle with vegetable salt.
5. Bake uncovered at 375 degrees for about 15 minutes, or until tender.

YIELDS: 4 SERVINGS

Nutritional breakdown: 4 grams protein, 16 grams carbohydrate, 7 grams fat
Serving portion: 1/4 recipe
Calories per serving: 135

Baked Onions

2 Spanish onions
2 tsps seasoned vegetable salt

1. Peel onions and slice in half.
2. Place each half on a foil square.
3. Sprinkle each half with 1/2 tsp vegetable salt.
4. Seal foil and bake at 350 degrees for 45 to 50 minutes, or barbecue on grill.

YIELDS: 4 SERVINGS

Nutritional breakdown: 4 grams protein, 28 grams carbohydrate, 0 grams fat
Serving portion: 1/2 onion
Calories per serving: 124

Use leftover vegetables from last night's dinner for today's lunch soup by running them through a blender with a clove of garlic and chicken broth.

Ratatouille

1/4 cup olive oil
1 large red onion, thinly sliced (1/2 cup)
4 garlic cloves, chopped fine
1 medium eggplant, washed and chunked
  (approximately 2 cups)
3 to 4 small zucchini, chunked
  (approximately 2 cups)
1 green bell pepper, chunked
3 to 4 large ripe tomatoes, cut into wedges
1/4 cup chopped fresh basil, or 4 tsps
  crushed dried basil
Salt and pepper to taste
1 lb fresh mushrooms, cut in half

1. In a large skillet, heat oil. Add onion and garlic; cook until transparent.
2. Add eggplant, zucchini, pepper, tomatoes, basil, and seasoning. Stir frequently until almost done.
3. When nearly ready, add mushrooms.
4. Cover and let sit until ready to serve.

YIELDS: 8 SERVINGS

Nutritional breakdown: 3 grams protein, 10 grams carbohydrate, 7 grams fat
Serving portion: 1/8 recipe
Calories per serving: 106
Recipe courtesy Terry Ganes

Squash Medley

This is one of the first recipes Jack taught me, and I've been converted to good, simple food ever since.

1 large zucchini (or 2 small, about 1 cup)
1 large summer squash (or 2 small, about 1 cup)
1 large gooseneck yellow squash (or 2 small, about 1 cup)
1 small onion, or 2 green onions
1 tbsp safflower oil

Chop the ingredients into bite-size pieces and sauté in safflower oil, keeping the ingredients crisp.

Variation:

Add 1/2 lb ground turkey, seasoning to taste (salt, pepper, garlic, onion powder), and sautéing until meat is cooked.

YIELDS: 2 SERVINGS

Nutritional breakdown: 3 grams protein, 13 grams carbohydrate, 7 grams fat
Serving portion: 1/2 recipe
Calories per serving: 111

Zucchini Halves

1 zucchini, 4 to 6 inches long
1 tsp safflower oil
1/4 tsp garlic powder
1/4 tsp vegetable seasoning

1. Slice zucchini in half lengthwise.
2. Using a pastry brush, lightly brush each cut half with safflower oil. Season with garlic powder and vegetable seasoning.
3. Place on a foil-covered baking sheet.
4. Broil approximately 8 to 10 inches from heat until tender and crisp.

YIELDS: 1 SERVING

Nutritional breakdown: 2 grams protein, 5 grams carbohydrate, 5 grams fat
Serving portion: 1 zucchini
Calories per serving: 63

Sweet Potatoes with Banana and Apples

4 medium sweet potatoes
2 medium bananas
1/4 cup orange juice
4 medium apples
1/2 cup honey
1/2 tsp cinnamon
2 tbsps safflower oil
1 tsp lemon juice
1/2 cup warm water

1. Cook potatoes until tender; cool, peel, and cut into 1-inch-thick slices.
2. Slice bananas and toss with orange juice.
3. Core apples and slice into 1/2-inch rings.
4. Mix together the honey, cinnamon, and oil.
5. Arrange potatoes, apples, and sliced bananas in alternate layers in an oiled baking dish. Sprinkle the honey mixture and lemon juice over each layer. Add water.
6. Cover, and bake at 375 degrees for 35 minutes.
7. Remove cover and bake another 10 minutes.

YIELDS: 6 SERVINGS

Nutritional breakdown: 2 grams protein, 65 grams carbohydrate, 5 grams fat
Serving portion: 1/6 recipe
Calories per serving: 300
Recipe courtesy Eleanor Vallée Hustedt

Old-fashioned Baked Beans

2 cups water
2 cups apple juice
1 1/2 cups dried kidney or soy beans (soak overnight)
2 tbsps dark honey
2 tomatoes, diced
1 tbsp dry mustard
1 tsp vegetable salt
1/2 cup boiling bean stock
1/2 tsp vinegar
1 tsp curry powder
1/2 cup finely minced onion

1. Bring water and apple juice to a boil and add beans slowly, so that boiling doesn't stop.
2. Reduce heat and cook until beans are almost tender. Drain beans, reserving liquid, and add remaining ingredients to beans, reserving 1 tablespoon tomato and 1 tablespoon onion for garnishing.
3. Place in an oiled baking dish and bake, covered, 2 to 3 hours in a 250-degree oven.
4. Uncover the last hour of cooking. If beans become dry, add a little of the reserved bean water.
5. Remove from oven, sprinkle on garnish, and serve.

YIELDS: 6 SERVINGS

Nutritional breakdown: 4 grams protein, 19 grams carbohydrate, 1 gram fat
Serving portion: 1/6 recipe
Calories per serving: 103

 # Brown and Wild Rice Casserole

1 cup uncooked wild rice
1 cup uncooked brown rice
1 cup dried currants
1/2 cup pine nuts, toasted
1/4 cup chopped Italian parsley
2 tbsps grated orange zest
1/4 cup olive oil
2 tbsps fresh orange juice
1/4 tsp freshly ground pepper
2 tbsps grated Parmesan cheese

1. Preheat oven to 350 degrees.
2. Cook rices according to package directions. Both rices should be just tender. Drain wild rice if necessary.
3. Combine both rices in a large bowl and add remaining ingredients except cheese.
4. Transfer to an ovenproof dish and bake covered until just heated through, 20 to 30 minutes.
5. Just before serving, sprinkle on Parmesan cheese.

YIELDS: 6 SERVINGS

Nutritional breakdown: 12 grams protein, 59 grams carbohydrate, 22 grams fat
Serving portion: 1/6 recipe
Calories per serving: 463
Recipe courtesy Lucy Thomas, Louisiana Pacific Corp.

Mushroom-Barley Pilaf

2 tbsps olive oil
1 onion, chopped fine
1 garlic clove, minced
4 cups water or chicken broth
4 medium mushrooms, thinly sliced
1 cup pearl barley
Salt and freshly ground black pepper to
  taste
1/4 cup chopped parsley

1. Heat olive oil over medium heat in a medium saucepan; sauté onion and garlic and cook until tender.
2. Add water or broth, mushrooms, and barley. Season to taste with salt and pepper.
3. Bring to a boil, reduce heat, and simmer about 45 minutes, or until barley is tender and liquid has been absorbed.
4. Just before serving, sprinkle with parsley.

YIELDS: 4 SERVINGS

Nutritional breakdown: 6 grams protein, 42 grams carbohydrate, 7 grams fat
Serving portion: 1/4 recipe
Calories per serving: 250
Recipe courtesy Liz Cardenas

 # Patricia's Lentil and Brown Rice Casserole

1 (14-oz) pkg lentils
1 cup uncooked brown rice
3 quarts distilled water
4 carrots, chopped
3 celery ribs, chopped
2 onions, diced
4 garlic cloves, chopped
2 tsps Bragg Liquid Aminos or soy sauce
1/4 tsp Italian herbs (oregano, basil, etc.)
2 tbsps olive oil
Tomatoes (optional)

1. Wash and drain lentils and rice. Place grains in a large iron or stainless steel pot. Add distilled water. Bring to a boil, reduce heat, and simmer for 30 minutes.
2. Add vegetables (except tomatoes) and seasonings and cook on low heat until done.
3. Just before serving, you may add fresh or canned whole tomatoes. Additional water may be used in cooking the grains to make this dish a soup.

YIELDS: 8 SERVINGS

Nutritional breakdown: 7 grams protein, 33 grams carbohydrate, 4 grams fat
Serving portion: 1/8 recipe
Calories per serving: 192
Recipe courtesy Patricia Bragg

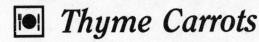 Potatoes LaLanne

1 medium potato
2 tsps safflower oil or any good vegetable oil
Seasoning to taste

1. Wash unskinned potato. Scrub carefully as though for baking. Then dry.
2. Slice potato crosswise in approximately 1/8-inch thickness. Dip each slice in a mixture of safflower oil and seasoning, according to taste. You may want to use garlic and/or onion powder.
3. Place each slice separately on a large sheet of foil (laid on a baking sheet). Place under broiler, which has been preheated for 5 minutes.
4. Broil 3 to 5 minutes, or until crispy brown. Flip the slices and brown the other side. Serve with meal or as a substitute for potato chips.

YIELDS: 1 SERVING

Nutritional breakdown: 3 grams protein, 34 grams carbohydrate, 9 grams fat
Serving portion: 1 potato
Calories per serving: 227

Thyme Carrots

1 carrot
1 tsp vegetable cooking oil
1/2 tsp thyme
1/4 tsp vegetable salt

1. Scrub carrot and cut into diagonal 1-inch slices.
2. Coat saucepan with oil. Sauté carrots for 3 to 4 minutes.
3. Sprinkle on thyme and salt. Cook for 1 to 2 minutes more, or until tender and crisp.

Variation:

Substitute ginger for thyme.

YIELDS: 1 SERVING

Nutritional breakdown: 1 gram protein, 8 grams carbohydrate, 5 grams fat
Serving portion: 1 carrot
Calories per serving: 74
Recipe courtesy Eileen Rorem

🔳 Stuffed Potatoes

2 medium baking potatoes
1/4 cup skim milk
2 eggs or egg substitutes
2 tbsps grated Parmesan cheese
2 tsps Dijon mustard
1 cup frozen chopped broccoli, thawed,
  drained, and finely chopped
1 green onion, minced
1 tsp thyme leaves
Salt and pepper, to taste

1. Scrub potatoes and prick with a fork. Bake potatoes at 400 degrees for 1 hour, or until tender when squeezed.
2. Cut each potato in half lengthwise. Scoop out pulp, leaving about a 1/4-inch shell. Arrange potato shells in a baking dish.
3. Beat pulp with skim milk, eggs, Parmesan cheese, and mustard until smooth. Stir in remaining ingredients. Mound filling into shells.
4. Return potatoes to oven and bake for 20 minutes, or until hot.

YIELDS: 4 SERVINGS

Nutritional breakdown: 8 grams protein, 21 grams carbohydrate, 4 grams fat
Serving portion: 1 stuffed half potato
Calories per serving: 146
Recipe courtesy Safeway, Inc., 1982

🔳 Oven Polenta

5 cups regular strength chicken broth
1 1/2 cups yellow cornmeal
1 small onion, chopped
4 tablespoons margarine, or 1/4 cup
  safflower oil
Jack cheese, shredded (optional)

1. In a shallow 9 x 12-inch baking dish, stir together the chicken broth, cornmeal, onion, and margarine.
2. Bake in a 350-degree oven until liquid is absorbed, 45 to 50 minutes.
3. Remove from oven and serve. Sprinkle lightly with shredded Jack cheese, if desired.

YIELDS: 6 SERVINGS

Nutritional breakdown: 5 grams protein, 10 grams carbohydrate, 10 grams fat
Serving portion: 1/6 recipe
Calories per serving: 153
Recipe courtesy Raechel Parker

Lima Bean Supreme

1 cup dried baby lima beans
1 onion, chopped
1 to 2 carrots, grated
1 green bell pepper, chopped
Seasoning to taste

1. Rinse and soak beans for 4 to 5 hours, or microwave for 15 to 20 minutes at full power, making certain beans are always covered with water. To cook beans, add more water to pot so that beans are amply covered.
2. Add chopped onion and cook until almost tender. Then add grated carrots and bell pepper. Season to taste. Cook until tender.

YIELDS: 3 CUPS

Nutritional breakdown: 5 grams protein, 21 grams carbohydrate, 0 grams fat
Serving portion: 1/2 cup
Calories per serving: 104

 # *Quick and Easy New Potatoes*

1 tbsp safflower oil
1/2 to 1 new potato, skin on
1/2 garlic clove, minced
1/4 cup chopped parsley

1. Brush oil over bottom of baking dish. Place potatoes in baking dish, then sprinkle on remaining ingredients, stirring to coat potatoes with oil, parsley, and garlic.
2. Bake at 350 degrees for 30 to 45 minutes, stirring again halfway through.

YIELDS: 1 SERVING

Nutritional breakdown: 4 grams protein, 35 grams carbohydrate, 14 grams fat
Serving portion: 1 potato
Calories per serving: 272

Fresh Green Beans with Almonds

1 1/2 lbs straight green beans
4 garlic cloves
1/2 tsp salt
1/2 tsp vegetable seasoning (unsalted)
1 cup water
1/4 cup slivered almonds
2 tsps safflower oil

1. Snip tips off beans and place in a 10-inch pan in an aligned arrangement.
2. Peel and slice garlic and sprinkle over beans. Add salt, vegetable seasoning, and water. Cook until tender.
3. Brown almonds in safflower oil.
4. Drain beans (save broth for future use in soup). Pour browned almonds over beans and serve.

YIELDS: 6 SERVINGS

Nutritional breakdown: 3 grams protein, 8 grams carbohydrate, 4 grams fat
Serving portion: 1/6 recipe
Calories per serving: 72
Recipe courtesy Ruth Allen

 # Cucumber Dill Sauce

1 cup chopped green onions
1 cup chicken broth
1 tbsp arrowroot
1 tbsp lemon juice
1 1/2 to 2 tsps dill weed
2 tbsps cooking oil (safflower, etc.)
1 medium cucumber, peeled and chopped fine

1. Mix all ingredients except cucumber in a blender.
2. Put mix into a saucepan and cook until thick. Add the cucumber and cook a minute or two. Pour hot over cooked vegetables, or serve with poached or steamed fish.

YIELDS: 1 3/4 CUPS

Nutritional breakdown: 2 grams protein, 5 grams carbohydrate, 4 grams fat
Serving portion: 1/4 cup
Calories per serving: 61

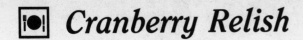 *Cranberry Relish*

1 quart fresh cranberries
2 oranges
4 apples
1 1/2 to 2 cups honey

1. Put all fruit into a food chopper or blender. Add honey. Mix well.
2. Store in a covered jar in a cool place.
3. Delicious served with turkey or chicken.

Hint:

Scoop out orange halves and use pulp in relish. Use shells as serving bowls.

YIELDS: 2 QUARTS

Nutritional breakdown: 0 grams protein, 6 grams carbohydrate, 0 grams fat
Serving portion: 1/4 cup
Calories per serving: 23

Purée pineapple and apple slices, and use as a substitute for butter.

Mother's Whole Wheat Bread

2 tsps salt
11 cups whole wheat flour, stone-ground
1 tbsp ground cinnamon
1/4 cup raisins
1/4 cup crushed walnuts
6 cups plus 5 tbsps warm water
2 pkgs active dry yeast
3 tbsps dark molasses

1. In a large bowl, mix the salt with the flour. Add cinammon, raisins, and walnuts. Stir to distribute ingredients evenly. Place in a 150-degree oven to warm flour.

2. In a coffee cup, pour 5 tablespoons warm water. Sprinkle active dry yeast on top of water. Allow to stand in a warm place for 2 minutes. Add molasses and set aside for 12 to 15 minutes, or until mixture begins to froth.

3. Remove bowl of flour from oven, pour in yeast mixture, and add 6 cups water. Mix by hand until ingredients are mixed evenly. Dough should be slightly tacky but should not stick to sides of bowl.

4. Distribute dough evenly into three 9x5-inch baking pans, sprayed with nonstick vegetable oil.

5. Place pans in a warm place, cover them with a towel or cloth, and allow to stand for 20 minutes, or until dough roughly doubles in size.

6. Bake in a preheated oven at 400 degrees, for 40 minutes.

7. Remove from pans and allow to cool on a rack.

YIELDS: 3 LOAVES (12 SLICES EACH)

Nutritional breakdown: 11 grams protein, 58 grams carbohydrate, 2 grams fat
Serving portion: 2 slices
Calories per serving: 276
Recipe courtesy Richard Benyo

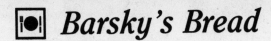 *Barsky's Bread*

4 cups wheat flour
1 tsp baking soda
1/2 tsp baking powder
1 tsp salt
1 tsp sugar
2 cups buttermilk

1. Stir flour with soda, baking powder, salt, and sugar until thoroughly mixed.
2. Make a well in the center of the mixture and add buttermilk.
3. Stir until well blended.
4. Knead gently on a floured board for 1 to 2 minutes until smooth.
5. Shape into 1 or 2 loaves and place on a baking sheet sprayed with nonstick vegetable oil. With the back of a knife, cut a deep cross in loaf and place immediately in a 400-degree oven. Bake 45 minutes, until golden.

YIELDS: 2 LOAVES (12 SLICES EACH)

Nutritional breakdown: 3 grams protein, 17 grams carbohydrate, 0 grams fat
Serving portion: 1 slice
Calories per serving: 85
Recipe courtesy Dr. Mark Rubenstein

Warm flour in a low heat oven (150 degrees) before baking with it for better rising.

▣ Sesame Crescents

1/2 cup cracked wheat
1 tbsp active dry yeast
1 cup warm water (110 degrees)
1/3 cup vegetable oil
1/2 cup honey
1 tsp salt
3/4 cup mashed potatoes, cooled (save cooking water)
1 cup potato water (110 degrees)
2 eggs, beaten
5 to 5 1/2 cups whole wheat flour
1 egg white, beaten
1/2 cup sesame seeds

1. To soften cracked wheat: cover with hot water in a small bowl and allow to stand until softened, 1 to 1 1/2 hours. Drain. Dissolve yeast in 1 cup warm water.

2. In a mixer bowl, combine oil, honey, salt, mashed potatoes, potato water, and beaten eggs. Add dissolved yeast and softened cracked wheat. Stir in 3 cups flour and beat at medium speed for 2 to 3 minutes, or 150 strokes with a spoon. Add remaining flour to form a firm dough that leaves the sides of the bowl.

3. Turn dough out onto a floured board and knead until smooth and elastic. Place kneaded dough in an oiled bowl, turning to oil top. Cover bowl and allow to rise in a warm place until doubled in bulk, about 1 hour. Punch down dough; shape and bake crescents (or other shaped rolls) according to the following directions for refrigerator rolls:

4. Place kneaded dough in a large oiled bowl, turning to oil top. Cover well and place in refrigerator. Punch dough down as it rises. When ready to use, allow to warm to room temperature. Divide dough into 6 equal portions. On a lightly floured board, roll out each portion into a 9-inch round, about 1/2 inch thick. Brush with beaten egg white and sprinkle with sesame seeds. Cut round into 6 wedges; roll up each wedge beginning at wide end. Brush tops with beaten egg white and sprinkle with sesame seeds. Place on oiled baking sheets with points under. Cover and allow to rise in a warm place until finger pressed into dough leaves a dent. Bake in a preheated 375-degree oven for 20 to 25 minutes, or until well browned.

YIELDS: 3 DOZEN CRESCENTS

Nutritional breakdown: 4 grams protein, 16 grams carbohydrate, 4 grams fat
Serving portion: 1 crescent
Calories per serving: 106

Easy French Bread

2 pkgs active dry yeast
2 cups plus 1/2 cup warm water (110 degrees)
3 tbsps honey
6 cups whole wheat pastry flour
3/4 cup fortified whey powder or nonfat dry milk
1 tbsp salt
2 tbsps polyunsaturated oil

1. Dissolve yeast in 1/2 cup warm water in a 1-quart bowl. Add honey and set aside to allow to bubble.
2. Combine all dry ingredients in a large bowl; mix well. Add 2 cups water and oil to yeast mixture and pour into dry ingredients.
3. Mix until smooth, adding 1/2 cup more flour if necessary to reach kneading consistency. Knead 3 minutes.
4. Divide dough in half; form 2 loaves and place on a greased cookie sheet. Cut 3 diagonal slashes across tops and let rise.
5. Bake at 450 degrees for 45 minutes. Remove from pan to cool on a rack.

YIELDS: 2 LOAVES (12 SLICES EACH)

Nutritional breakdown: 9 grams protein, 50 grams carbohydrate, 3 grams fat
Serving portion: 2 slices
Calories per serving: 253
Recipe courtesy The Whey Lovers' Cookbook *by Christina Dillane and Susan Dusharme*

Desserts

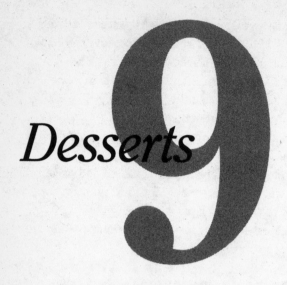

▣ *Reliable Rice Pudding*

12 oz brown rice, cooked
1 to 1 1/2 cups mashed tofu
3/4 cup nonfat dry milk or whey powder
3 tbsps honey
1/2 tsp cinnamon
1/8 tsp cloves
1/4 cup raisins
1 tsp safflower oil
3 tbsps granola

1. Combine rice, tofu, milk, honey, spices, and raisins in a large bowl. Mix well.
2. Coat a quart-size baking dish or bowl with oil. Spoon in tofu mixture. Sprinkle with granola.
3. Bake in a preheated 350-degree oven 45 minutes, or until set.

YIELDS: 6 SERVINGS

Nutritional breakdown: 14 grams protein, 42 grams carbohydrate, 8 grams fat
Serving portion: 1/6 recipe
Calories per serving: 283

When cooking rice, cook extra and freeze in serving-size bags for later use. Just steam and serve.

Natural Banana Pudding

1 ripe banana
1 tsp honey
1/2 tsp lemon juice

1. Mash banana with a fork and add honey and lemon juice.
2. Garnish with strawberries or fruit in season.

Variation:

Freeze ripe banana. Chop in a food processor with honey and lemon juice.

YIELDS: 1 SERVING

Nutritional breakdown: 1 gram protein, 33 grams carbohydrate, 9 grams fat
Serving portion: 1 banana
Calories per serving: 122

 # *Basic Custard*

4 eggs, slightly beaten, or egg substitutes
3/4 to 1 1/2 cups honey (depending on taste)
2 1/2 cups skim milk
1/2 tsp salt
1/2 tsp vanilla extract
Nutmeg (optional: before baking, you may
  sprinkle on top)

Mix all ingredients except nutmeg and oven poach at 350 degrees until a knife comes out clean from center of custard. (To oven poach, set individual cups or baking dish in a larger baking pan with about 1/2 inch of water.)

YIELDS: 6 SERVINGS

Nutritional breakdown: 8 grams protein, 51 grams carbohydrate, 4 grams fat
Serving portion: 1/6 recipe
Calories per serving: 260

▣ *Tropical Sherbet*

1 cup fresh or canned pineapple,
  unsweetened
1/2 cup low-fat yogurt
1 ripe banana
1 tbsp honey
2 tbsps fresh lemon juice

1. Process all ingredients in a blender and pour into an ice cube tray. Freeze.
2. When ready to serve, reprocess in blender until mixture is soft and creamy.

Variation:

Papaya and mango may be added.

YIELDS: 4 SERVINGS

Nutritional breakdown: 3 grams protein, 20 grams carbohydrate, 1 gram fat
Serving portion: 1/2 cup
Calories per serving: 100

▣ *Boysenberry Granité (Sherbet)*

3 lbs boysenberries, puréed in a food
  processor and strained through a fine
  strainer (should yield about 6 cups liquid)
3/4 cup honey or apple concentrate
Good squeeze of lemon juice

Put all ingredients into an ice cream maker to mix, then freeze.

YIELDS: 12 SERVINGS

Nutritional breakdown: 1 gram protein, 31 grams carbohydrate, 0 grams fat
Serving portion: 1/12 recipe (about 1/2 cup)
Calories per serving: 123

Light Strawberry Ice Cream

1 pint strawberries
1/2 cup honey or apple concentrate
2 cups canned evaporated skim milk
Juice of 1 lemon

1. Crush strawberries in a food processor after adding honey or apple concentrate.
2. Add skim milk and lemon and process until blended.
3. Freeze.

YIELDS: 8 SERVINGS

Nutritional breakdown: 5 grams protein, 28 grams carbohydrate, 0 grams fat
Serving portion: 1/8 recipe
Calories per serving: 132
Recipe courtesy Georgiene Malloy

 # *Cinnamon Apples*

1/4 cup frozen apple concentrate
1/4 cup cranberry juice
1 tsp cinnamon
4 cooking apples
1/2 cup raisins
1 lemon, sliced into 1/8-inch rounds

1. Whip both juices and cinnamon together.
2. Core apples and place upright in a 4-inch square baking dish. Stuff with raisins. Pour juice mixture over apples. Place a lemon slice on each apple.
3. Bake in a preheated 350-degree oven.
4. After 30 minutes, spoon sauce over apples.
5. Return to oven for 10 additional minutes.

YIELDS: 4 SERVINGS

Nutritional breakdown: 1 gram protein, 43 grams carbohydrate, 0 grams fat
Serving portion: 1 apple
Calories per serving: 165

Poached Pears in Raspberry Sauce

3 firm ripe pears
8 oz frozen raspberries, puréed and strained
1/2 cup pineapple juice, unsweetened
1 tsp lemon juice
2 tbsp frozen apple concentrate

1. Quarter and core pears, leaving skins on.
2. Combine raspberries, pineapple juice, lemon juice, and apple concentrate in a saucepan and bring to a boil.
3. Add pears, reduce heat, and cook approximately 20 minutes.
4. Chill and serve.

YIELDS: 6 SERVINGS

Nutritional breakdown: 1 gram protein, 29 grams carbohydrate, 0 grams fat
Serving portion: 1/2 pear
Calories per serving: 114

 # Bananas à L'Orange

4 firm bananas
1 orange
1/4 tsp rum extract (optional)
2 tbsps raisins
2 tbsps chopped nuts

1. Slice bananas in half lengthwise. Place in a baking dish.
2. Grate peel of orange; reserve. Halve orange and squeeze or press to remove juice.
3. Combine orange juice, orange peel, and rum extract; pour over bananas. Sprinkle with raisins.
4. Bake in a 400-degree oven for 15 minutes, or until tender. Top with nuts. Serve hot.

YIELDS: 4 SERVINGS

Nutritional breakdown: 2 grams protein, 35 grams carbohydrate, 3 grams fat
Serving portion: 1 banana
Calories per serving: 160
Recipe courtesy Safeway, Inc., 1982

Jellied Fruit

2 envelopes unflavored gelatin, or 1 bar
  agar-agar
1/2 cup boiling water
2 1/2 cups fruit juice
1 cup crushed fruit or mandarin orange
  sections

1. Place gelatin in a medium bowl. Slowly stir in boiling water, stirring until dissolved.
2. Add fruit juice and mix well.
3. Add fruit. Pour into a serving dish. Chill until firm and serve.

YIELDS: 8 SERVINGS

Nutritional breakdown: 2 grams protein, 12 grams carbohydrate, 0 grams fat
Serving portion: 1/2 cup
Calories per serving: 52

Pleasing Peach Meringues

1 cup dried apricots
1 cup water
1/4 cup honey
1 tbsp tapioca
3 or 4 fresh peaches, or a 16-oz can of
  unsweetened peaches
8 meringue mounds (see recipe on next
  page)

1. Purée apricots, water, honey, and tapioca in a blender.
2. Let stand for 5 minutes.
3. Put into a saucepan and cook and stir over medium heat until mixture comes to a full boil.
4. Remove from heat and allow to cool slightly.
5. Place 1/2 peach in the center of each meringue. Pour puréed fruit over.

YIELDS: 8 SERVINGS

Nutritional breakdown: 2 grams protein, 18 grams carbohydrate, 1 gram fat
Serving portion: 1 peach meringue
Calories per serving: 82

Meringue Mounds

3 egg whites
1/4 tsp cream of tartar
1/2 tsp vanilla extract
2 tbsps honey

1. Preheat oven to 275 degrees.
2. Use parchment paper or line a baking sheet with plain brown paper. (Hint: use a grocery bag).
3. Beat egg whites until foamy. Sprinkle on cream of tartar and continue beating.
4. Combine vanilla and honey. Gradually add to egg whites, beating until whites are stiff.
5. Spoon onto baking sheet in mounds. Make a depression in each. Bake about 1 hour, until dry and creamy in color.
6. Allow to cool, then carefully remove and store in an airtight container until ready for use.

YIELDS: 8 SHELLS

Nutritional breakdown: 1 gram protein, 5 grams carbohydrate, 0 grams fat
Serving portion: 1 shell
Calories per serving: 24

12-Minute Oatmeal Cookies

2/3 cup safflower oil
1 1/2 cups honey
1 egg
1/4 cup orange juice (or use 1/2 cup unsweetened apple juice)
1 tsp vanilla extract
3 cups quick-cooking oats, uncooked
1 cup whole wheat flour (you may combine with wheat germ)
1 tsp salt
1/2 tsp baking soda

1. Preheat oven to 350 degrees.
2. Beat together oil, honey, egg, juice, and vanilla until creamy. Add remaining ingredients; mix well.
3. Drop by rounded teaspoonfuls onto a greased cookie sheet.
4. Bake for 12 to 15 minutes.

Variation:

Add chopped nuts, raisins, or carob chips.

YIELDS: 4 DOZEN COOKIES

Nutritional breakdown: 4 grams protein, 34 grams carbohydrate, 7 grams fat
Serving portion: 2 cookies
Calories per serving: 215

Orange-Apricot Cookies

1 cup all-purpose flour
3/4 cup whole wheat flour
1/4 cup sugar
2 tsps baking powder
1/2 tsp cinnamon
1/4 tsp salt
3/4 cup dried apricots, chopped
1/2 cup orange juice, fresh
1/4 cup vegetable oil
1 tsp grated orange rind
1 egg, beaten

1. Preheat oven to 375 degrees.
2. Mix dry ingredients thoroughly. Add remaining ingredients. Mix well.
3. Drop dough by teaspoonful onto an ungreased baking sheet, about 1 inch apart.
4. Bake about 11 minutes, or until lightly browned.
5. Remove from baking sheet while still warm.
6. Cool on a rack.

YIELDS: 4 DOZEN COOKIES

Nutritional breakdown: 1 gram protein, 5 grams carbohydrate, 1 gram fat
Serving portion: 1 cookie
Calories per serving: 37
Recipe courtesy Safeway, Inc., 1990

Fruity Oat Bars

1 (6-oz) pkg mixed dried fruit, diced (1 1/3 cups)
3/4 cup water
1/4 tsp cinnamon
1 1/4 cups Quaker Oats (quick or old-fashioned, uncooked)
1/3 cup firmly packed brown sugar
1/4 cup all-purpose flour
4 tbsps margarine, melted

1. Heat oven to 350 degrees.
2. In a small saucepan, combine fruit, water, and cinnamon. Cook over low heat 10 minutes, stirring constantly, or until almost all liquid is absorbed. Remove from heat; cover. Set aside.
3. Combine oats, brown sugar, and flour. Add margarine; mix well until crumbly. Reserve 1/3 cup oat mixture; press remaining mixture onto the bottom of an 8- or 9-inch baking pan. Bake 10 to 15 minutes, or until golden brown.
4. Spread fruit filling evenly over base; sprinkle with reserved 1/3 cup oat mixture, patting lightly. Bake 20 minutes, or until topping is golden brown. Cool; cut into bars. Store loosely covered.

YIELDS: 9 SERVINGS

Nutritional breakdown: 2 grams protein, 31 grams carbohydrate, 5 grams fat
Serving portion: 1 bar cookie
Calories per serving: 180
Recipe courtesy Quaker Oats Company

Chris's Kringles

1/2 cup quick-cooking oats, uncooked
1/2 cup whole wheat flour
1 tsp cinnamon
1 tsp allspice
1/4 tsp nutmeg
1/2 tsp cloves
1/2 tsp baking soda
3/4 cup raisins
1 tsp vanilla extract
1 tbsp honey
2 tbsps light vegetable oil
2/3 cup unsweetened applesauce
1 unbeaten egg

1. Combine dry ingredients.
2. Add other ingredients and mix well.
3. Use a teaspoon to drop batter onto a lightly oiled cookie sheet, or use a nonstick spray.
4. Bake at 350 degrees for 15 minutes, or until light brown.

Hint:

If you like, substitute 2 packages of artificial sweetener (equivalent to 4 teaspoons sugar) in place of honey.

YIELDS: 2 DOZEN SMALL COOKIES

Nutritional breakdown: 4 grams protein, 33 grams carbohydrate, 6 grams fat
Serving portion: 4 cookies
Calories per serving: 194
Recipe courtesy Living Lean by Choosing More, by Cheryl Jennings-Sauer, MA, RD, LD (Taylor Publishing, 1989)

Banana Oatmeal Cookies

3 bananas
1/3 cup salad oil
2 cups quick-cooking oats, uncooked
1 to 1 1/2 cups chopped walnuts
1 tsp vanilla extract
3/4 tsp salt

1. In a large bowl, mash bananas and add other ingredients.
2. Drop by rounded tablespoons onto an ungreased cookie sheet.
3. Bake at 350 degrees for 20 to 25 minutes. Cool on a wire rack.

YIELDS: 2 1/2 DOZEN COOKIES

Nutritional breakdown: 2 grams protein, 6 grams carbohydrate, 5 grams fat
Serving portion: 1 cookie
Calories per serving: 76
Recipe courtesy Safeway, Inc., 1984

Carolyn's English Tea Bread

6 Indian tea bags
3 cups boiling water
2 cups golden raisins
2 cups dark raisins
3 eggs, or 5 egg whites
1 1/2 cups honey
3 tsps baking powder
3 tsps allspice
4 cups whole wheat pastry flour

1. Make tea with tea bags and 3 cups of boiling water. Allow to cool and then add all the raisins. Let soak for 2 to 3 hours (or better, overnight).
2. Beat the eggs to a light froth and add the honey gradually. Add the fruited tea and mix lightly. Add the baking powder and allspice and flour and mix lightly.
3. Spoon the mixture into 3 bread tins and bake for 1 3/4 hours at 300 degrees.
4. Remove from oven and let cool on a wire rack. Glaze the tops with melted honey before serving.

YIELDS: 3 LOAVES (12 SLICES EACH)

Nutritional breakdown: 3 grams protein, 35 grams carbohydrate, 0 grams fat
Serving portion: 1 slice
Calories per serving: 143
Recipe courtesy Carolyn Katzin

Date and Nut Squares

3 egg whites
1/3 cup honey
1/2 tsp vanilla extract
1/2 cup flour
1/2 tsp baking powder
1 cup chopped walnuts
1 1/2 cups finely chopped dates

1. Beat egg whites until foamy. Beat in honey and vanilla. Mix in remaining ingredients.
2. Put into an oiled and floured 8-inch square pan and bake at 375 degrees for 25 to 30 minutes, or until top has a dull crust.
3. Cut into squares and cool. Remove from pan.

YIELDS: 12 SERVINGS

Nutritional breakdown: 3 grams protein, 29 grams carbohydrate, 4 grams fat
Serving portion: 1 square
Calories per serving: 154

▣ *Light 'n' Luscious Cheesecake*

3/4 cup graham cracker crumbs (about 2 oz)
2 tbsps margarine, melted
I cup low-fat cottage cheese
I (8-oz) container plain low-fat yogurt
I (8-oz) pkg light cream cheese
1/2 cup sugar
2 tsps grated orange peel
2 tsps vanilla extract
2 egg whites

1. In small bowl, combine graham cracker crumbs and margarine. Pat into the bottom of an 8-inch springform pan. Bake in a 350-degree oven for 10 minutes. Lower oven temperature to 325 degrees.
2. Place cottage cheese in blender container. Cover and blend on high speed 2 minutes, or until smooth. Add yogurt, cream cheese, sugar, orange peel, and vanilla; blend until smooth.
3. Add egg whites; blend until well mixed. Pour into baked crust.
4. Bake in a 325-degree oven for 30 minutes.
5. Turn off oven. Leave cheesecake in oven with door ajar 30 minutes.
6. Cool on a wire rack. Refrigerate several hours, or until thoroughly chilled.
7. Before serving, remove side of pan. If desired, serve with orange slices.

YIELDS: 10 SERVINGS

Nutritional breakdown: 7 grams protein, 17 grams carbohydrate, 9 grams fat
Serving portion: 1/10 recipe
Calories per serving: 180
Recipe courtesy Mazola corn oil

In whipping egg whites, the highest volume is achieved by using eggs at room temperature.

Jewel Fruit Tart

1 cup graham cracker crumbs
3 tbsps diet margarine, melted
2 cups plain nonfat yogurt
5 tbsps sugar
2 tbsps all-purpose flour
1 egg
1 egg white
1/2 tsp grated orange rind
1/2 tsp vanilla extract
2 to 3 cups sliced fresh fruits
3 tbsps sugar-reduced orange marmalade,
  put through a sieve

1. Combine crumbs and margarine. Press on the bottom and sides of a 10-inch pie plate or tart pan. Bake in a 350-degree oven for 5 minutes.
2. While crust bakes, combine yogurt, sugar, flour, egg, egg white, orange rind, and vanilla in a bowl; blend well. Pour into crust.
3. Return to oven and bake for 20 minutes, or until set.
4. Remove and cool.
5. Arrange fruit, overlapping, on tart. Brush with sieved marmalade.
6. Refrigerate until ready to serve.

YIELDS: 8 SERVINGS

Nutritional breakdown: 6 grams protein, 29 grams carbohydrate, 4 grams fat
Serving portion: 1/8 pie
Calories per serving: 173
Recipe courtesy Safeway, Inc., 1990

Natural Apple Candy

1 1/2 envelopes unflavored gelatin
1/4 cup cold water
1 cup unsweetened applesauce
1/2 (12-oz) can frozen apple juice
  concentrate
1/2 cup chopped walnuts
1/4 tsp cinnamon

1. Dissolve gelatin in cold water and set aside.
2. Combine applesauce and apple concentrate. Cook until a candy thermometer reaches 200 degrees.
3. Remove from heat, add gelatin, and stir well.
4. Add chopped walnuts and cinnamon.
5. Pour into vegetable-sprayed 8x8-inch baking dish.
6. Let stand until firm and cut into 32 rectangles.

YIELDS: 16 SERVINGS

Nutritional breakdown: 2 grams protein, 4 grams carbohydrate, 2 grams fat
Serving portion: 2 rectangles
Calories per serving: 38

Richard's Apple Pie

1/2 cup sugar
2 tbsps flour
1 tbsp cinnamon
1 tbsp nutmeg
1/8 tsp salt
4 large tart apples
Unbaked whole wheat pie crust (see
  following recipe)
2 tbsps raisins
1 tbsp margarine

1. Into a large bowl combine sugar, flour, cinnamon, nutmeg, and salt. Stir until ingredients are blended evenly.

2. Peel, core, and slice apples into the bowl, using a tablespoon to sprinkle sugar mixture over apple slices. As apple pieces are covered with mixture, place into pie crust, layering as you go. Fill shell with tightly packed and layered coated apple slices. Sprinkle remaining mixture over exposed apples. Sprinkle on raisins. Add small dabs of margarine evenly around apples.

3. Bake in a preheated 375-degree oven for 40 minutes.

YIELDS: 8 SERVINGS

Nutritional breakdown: 4 grams protein, 37 grams carbohydrate, 10 grams fat
Serving portion: 1/8 pie
Calories per serving (including crust): 245
Recipe courtesy Richard Benyo

Whole Wheat Pie Crust

Ice cubes
Water
1 1/2 cups whole wheat pastry flour
1/4 tsp salt
1/3 cup unsaturated vegetable oil

1. Put ice cubes in a glass of water. Set aside.

2. Sift flour and salt together. Slowly add oil and 3 to 4 tablespoons ice water, moving flour with a fork.

3. Form mixture into a smooth ball and roll out between sheets of wax paper, carefully forming a circle.

4. Fit into pie pan and flute edges. Prick bottom and sides.

5. Bake in a preheated 375-degree oven for 15 to 20 minutes, or until firm and brown.

YIELDS: 9-INCH PIE CRUST

◧ *Apple Bertie*

3 apples (Jonathan, Delicious, Rome)
2 tbsps flour
1/4 cup quick-cooking oats, uncooked
1 pkg NutraSweet
1/2 tsp cinnamon and/or nutmeg, allspice
1/2 cup frozen apple juice concentrate
1/2 tsp canola or vegetable oil

1. Wash and core apples. Dice them, peeled or unpeeled.
2. Combine flour, oats, NutraSweet, and spice in a gallon-size plastic bag.
3. Add apple pieces and shake to coat.
4. Pour apple juice concentrate into an oiled or vegetable-sprayed baking dish (8x8 inches).
5. Add coated diced apples. Cover dish and bake 20 minutes at 375 degrees.
6. Remove cover and continue baking 15 minutes more, or until well done.

Variation:

Sprinkle 1/2 cup diced walnuts or hulled sunflower seeds on apples before baking.
May also be prepared in 4 individual ramekins (baking dishes).

YIELDS: 4 SERVINGS

Nutritional breakdown: 1 gram protein, 28 grams carbohydrate, 1 gram fat
Serving portion: 1/4 recipe
Calories per serving: 121
Recipe courtesy Bertie Gorman

To make pie crusts, roll them between two pieces of waxed paper. Dampen the surface on which you will be rolling the crusts so that the waxed paper will not slip.

Frosted Baby Cakes

1/4 cup orange juice
1/4 cup carob powder
1 cup powdered milk or soya powder
1 tbsp safflower oil
1 tbsp hot water
1 tsp vanilla extract
1/4 cup honey
Mini-rice cakes

1. Combine all ingredients except rice cakes and beat with an electric mixer.
2. Use as frosting on mini-rice cakes, using 1 teaspoon frosting, and garnish with a slice of kiwi, strawberry, or banana.

Variation:

Substitute hot coffee for orange juice.

Hint:

For smooth consistency, use powdered milk and powdered carob, not granules.

YIELDS: 1 CUP

Nutritional breakdown: 2 grams protein, 9 grams carbohydrate, 3 grams fat
Serving portion: 3 teaspoons frosting
Calories per serving: 69
Calories per 3 mini-rice cakes: 25

Old-Fashioned Brownies

1/4 cup safflower oil
1 cup honey
2 eggs or egg substitutes
1 tsp vanilla extract
1/3 cup carob powder
2/3 cup oat flour or whole wheat pastry
  flour
1/8 tsp salt
1/2 cup chopped walnuts

1. Combine oil, honey, eggs, and vanilla.
2. Add dry ingredients, mixing well; stir in nuts.
3. Bake in an 8 x 8-inch square baking dish (prepared with vegetable spray).
4. Bake approximately 45 minutes at 350 degrees; remove from oven. Brownies should be moist.

YIELDS: 24 BARS

Nutritional breakdown: 3 grams protein, 31 grams carbohydrate, 8 grams fat
Serving portion: 2 bars
Calories per serving: 200

Strawberry Cake

Cake:

1 cup whole wheat pastry flour (sifted)
1/2 cup honey
3 tbsps nonfat dry milk powder (instant)
1 tsp baking powder
1/8 tsp salt
3 tbsps safflower oil
1 tsp vanilla extract
1/2 cup water
2 egg whites

1. Combine flour, honey, powdered milk, baking powder, and salt in a large mixing bowl; stir well.
2. Combine oil, vanilla, and water using a wire whisk. Stir into flour mixture until the dry mixture is moistened.
3. Beat egg whites at high speed with an electric mixer until stiff, then fold into batter.
4. Spoon batter into a 9-inch springform pan that has been coated with vegetable spray.
5. Bake at 350 degrees for 25 to 30 minutes, or until you can insert a wooden pick into the center and remove clean.
6. Remove cake from pan and cool on a wire rack.
7. Place cake on a serving plate and decorate with topping and strawberries.

Nutritional breakdown (for cake only): 3 grams protein, 21 grams carbohydrate, 4 grams fat
Serving portion: 1/10 recipe
Calories: 132

Topping:

1/3 cup orange juice
1 envelope unflavored gelatin
1/2 cup cold water
1/2 cup honey
1/4 cup lemon juice
1/3 cup instant nonfat dry milk powder
2 egg whites
4 cups fresh strawberries (hulled)

1. Place orange juice in a small container and freeze for 25 minutes, or until a 1/8-inch layer of ice forms on surface.
2. Sprinkle gelatin over cold water in a small saucepan; let stand for 1 minute. Cook over low heat, stirring until gelatin dissolves.
3. Add honey and lemon juice. Chill until the consistency of unbeaten egg white.
4. Add milk powder to partially frozen orange juice. Beat at high speed with an electric mixer for 5 minutes, or until stiff peaks form.
5. Beat egg whites in a small bowl at high speed with electric mixer until soft peaks form. Fold egg whites and whipped milk mixture into gelatin mixture.

YIELDS: 1 CAKE WITH TOPPING; 10 SERVINGS

Nutritional breakdown (cake and topping): 5 grams protein, 37 grams carbohydrate, 4 grams fat
Serving portion: 1/10 recipe
Calories per serving: 203

Upside-Down Gingerbread

1 1/2 cups whole wheat pastry flour
1 level tsp baking soda
1/2 tsp salt
1 tsp ginger
1/2 tsp cinnamon
1/2 tsp nutmeg
1/4 cup unsaturated vegetable oil
1/3 cup frozen apple juice concentrate
1/3 cup honey
1/2 cup plain nonfat yogurt
1 large egg
1 medium apple
1/2 cup frozen apple juice concentrate

1. Measure all the dry ingredients into a large bowl and mix well with a fork.
2. Measure all the wet ingredients into a 2-cup measure and mix well, in the cup.
3. Add wet ingredients to dry ingredients and mix until uniform.
4. Core, peel, and slice apple.
5. Pour 1/2 cup apple concentrate into an oiled 8-inch square pan.
6. Arrange apple slices in concentrate.
7. Cover with batter.
8. Bake in a preheated 375-degree oven for 35 to 40 minutes. Test for doneness; cut right in the pan, or serve upside down.

YIELDS: 12 SERVINGS

Nutritional breakdown: 3 grams protein, 25 grams carbohydrate, 5 grams fat
Serving portion: 1/12 recipe
Calories per serving: 155

Prize Carrot Cake

1 1/2 cups whole wheat pastry flour (sifted)
2 tsps baking powder
1 tsp baking soda
1/2 tsp salt
1 tsp cinnamon
3/4 cup unsaturated vegetable oil
1 cup unsweetened crushed pineapple
3/4 cup honey
3 eggs, or 4 egg whites
2 1/2 cups grated raw carrots
1 cup finely chopped nuts (your choice)

1. Sift together flour, baking powder, baking soda, salt, and cinnamon.
2. Make a well in the center of dry ingredients.
3. Add oil, pineapple, honey, and eggs. Mix thoroughly. Add grated carrots and mix well; then mix in chopped nuts.
4. Pour into a well-oiled 9 x 12-inch baking pan.
5. Bake at 325 degrees for approximately 45 minutes.

YIELDS: 12 SERVINGS

Nutritional breakdown: 6 grams protein, 34 grams carbohydrate, 20 grams fat
Serving portion: 1/12 recipe
Calories per serving: 323

Drinks

10

▣ *Fruit Spritzers*

1 cup fruit juice
1 cup fruit
1 cup sparkling water
or
2 cups fruit juice
1 cup sparkling water
or
1 cup fruit
2 cups sparkling water

Using any fresh fruit (melons, berries, peaches, bananas, etc.) and any fruit juice, combine ingredients at slow speed in a blender for a refreshing summer drink.

YIELDS: 3 CUPS

Nutritional breakdown: 1 gram protein, 23 grams carbohydrate, 0 grams fat
Serving portion: 1 1/2 cups
Calories per serving: 98

Hard lemons can be rejuvenated by soaking them overnight in lukewarm water.

Alfalfa Tea

1 cup alfalfa seeds
2 quarts cold water

1. Mix seeds and water. Bring to a boil in a pot.
2. Cool. Strain and store in a glass jar in refrigerator.
3. Use 1/4 to 1/2 glass of this extract, then fill glass with water. Serve either hot or cold, with or without honey. Add mint leaves (optional).

YIELDS: 2 QUARTS

Nutritional breakdown: 0 grams protein, 0 grams carbohydrate, 0 grams fat
Serving portion: 1 cup
Calories per serving: 1

Lemon and Barley Tea

Recipe is of Old English extraction

10 cups water
1/2 cup pearl barley
2 lemons, cut into quarters

1. Bring water and barley to a boil and add quartered lemon.
2. Simmer with lid on pan for 1 hour.
3. When completely cooled, strain into a container. Serve hot or cold.
4. Can be sweetened by adding honey.

YIELDS: 10 CUPS

Nutritional breakdown: 1 gram protein, 9 grams carbohydrate, 0 grams fat
Serving portion: 1 cup
Calories per serving: 38

Lemon-Orange Spicy Drink

3 oranges
2 lemons
6 cups water
Stick of cinnamon
I tsp whole cloves
I cup honey

1. Squeeze the juice of oranges and lemons and set aside.
2. Coarsely chop the rinds and combine with water, spices, and honey in a 2- or 3-quart saucepan.
3. Boil for 5 minutes and strain into a pitcher. Discard rinds and spices.
4. Let cool and add the juices. Chill.

YIELDS: 8 CUPS

Nutritional breakdown: I gram protein, 42 grams carbohydrate, 0 grams fat
Serving portion: I cup
Calories per serving: 159

 # *Bran Broth*

I cup bran flakes
2 cups cold water
I cup hot water
Lemon juice

1. Combine bran flakes and cold water. Allow to soak for several hours or overnight.
2. Strain liquid into a bowl, then pour hot water through the bran flakes and strain into the bowl.
3. Add a few drops of lemon juice to the liquid or broth. Store in refrigerator.
4. This broth contains the water soluble nutrients of bran. It can be used in hot or cold beverages, in sauces or soups, or as the liquid in baking bread. Use the remaining soaked bran flakes in cereals or bread.

YIELDS: 3 CUPS

Nutritional breakdown: 2 grams protein, 13 grams carbohydrate, 0 grams fat
Serving portion: I cup
Calories per serving: 54

Strawberry Buttermilk Cooler

2 cups buttermilk
1 cup fresh or frozen unsweetened
  strawberries

Mix in a blender at slow speed. Serve chilled.

YIELDS: 3 CUPS

Nutritional breakdown: 9 grams protein, 17 grams carbohydrate, 2 grams fat
Serving portion: 1 1/2 cups
Calories per serving: 121

 # *Skinny Strawberry Shake*

2 cups fresh or frozen unsweetened
  strawberries
1 cup ice cubes
1 1/2 cups apple juice
Dash of cinnamon

Place ingredients in a blender. Blend at medium speed, or until smooth.

YIELDS: 4 CUPS

Nutritional breakdown: 0 grams protein, 21 grams carbohydrate, 0 grams fat
Serving portion: 1 1/3 cups
Calories per serving: 80

 # *Refreshing Pear Shake*

1 medium pear, peeled, cored and cut into
  chunks
1 tbsp lemon juice
1 (5.5-oz) can apple juice
3/4 cup skim milk
3/4 cup crushed ice
Dash of cinnamon and nutmeg

Blend at medium speed until smooth.

YIELDS: 2 CUPS

Nutritional breakdown: 4 grams protein, 32 grams carbohydrate, 1 gram fat
Serving portion: 1 cup
Calories per serving: 142
Recipe courtesy Liz Cardenas

Emergency Prune Juice

1/2 box pitted prunes (6 oz)
1 1/2 cups water
1 tbsp lemon juice

Place ingredients in a blender. Blend on medium speed until of smooth enough consistency to drink.

YIELDS: 2 CUPS

Nutritional breakdown: 1 gram protein, 27 grams carbohydrate, 0 grams fat
Serving portion: 1/2 cup
Calories per serving: 103

 # *Fruit Teas*

Leaves from any vined berry (blackberry, raspberry, etc.)

1. Wash leaves thoroughly and pat dry.
2. Freeze on a baking sheet.
3. Once frozen, store in plastic freezer bags.
4. Steep a few leaves in boiling water or add to regular tea to enhance flavor.

Nutritional breakdown: 0 grams protein, 0 grams carbohydrate, 0 grams fat
Serving portion: 6 leaves per pot of tea
Calories per serving: 1

 # *Banana Yogurt Flip*

1 cup plain or fruited low-fat yogurt
1 ripe medium banana
1/2 cup orange juice, apple juice, or
   pineapple juice
1/4 cup Quaker Oats (quick or
   old-fashioned, uncooked)
1 tbsp honey
1/8 tsp nutmeg (optional)
1/2 cup crushed ice, or 4 to 5 ice cubes

Put all ingredients in a blender or food processor. Blend on high speed about 1 minute, or until smooth.

YIELDS: 2 CUPS

Nutritional information: 7 grams protein, 54 grams carbohydrate, 1 gram fat
Serving portion: 1 cup
Calories per serving: 230
Recipe courtesy Quaker Oats Company

Lemonade Blush

6 cups cran-apple juice, unsweetened
1 cup lemon juice, unstrained
1/2 cup honey
Fresh mint sprigs

1. Combine both fruit juices.
2. Warm honey until it flows easily, then add to fruit juices, stirring until it dissolves.
3. Serve over ice. Garnish with a mint sprig.

YIELDS: 7 1/2 CUPS

Nutritional breakdown: 0 grams protein, 42 grams carbohydrate, 0 grams fat
Serving portion: 1/8 recipe
Calories per serving: 160
Recipe courtesy Leone Lyons

Be-Fit Beverage

1/2 medium carrot
1 celery rib
1/2 small onion
1 small zucchini
1 small green bell pepper
1 tsp vegetable salt
1 cup tomato juice
1 cup water
1 cup clam juice, or 1 (6-oz) can minced clams
1/2 cucumber, seeded

1. Place all vegetables except cucumber in a saucepan.
2. Sprinkle with seasoning, cover, and steam until tender.
3. Place tomato juice, water, clam juice, and seeded cucumber in blender; add steamed vegetables and liquefy. Seasonings may be added to taste.

Variation:

If you own a juicer, juice all vegetables (leave out onion).

YIELDS: 4 CUPS

Nutritional breakdown: 4 grams protein, 6 grams carbohydrate, less than 1 gram fat
Serving portion: 3/4 cup
Calories per serving: 36

Pineapple Mint Julep

4 fresh mint sprigs
1/4 cup honey
1/2 cup fresh lemon juice
1 1/4 cups pineapple juice, unsweetened

1. Wash mint leaves in a large bowl and bruise with a spoon; cover with honey. Add lemon juice and let stand about 15 minutes.
2. Add pineapple juice and mix.
3. Pour over ice in a pitcher or tall glasses. Garnish with sprigs of mint.

YIELDS: 2 CUPS

Nutritional breakdown: 0 grams protein, 37 grams carbohydrate, 0 grams fat
Serving portion: 1/3 cup
Calories per serving: 144
Recipe courtesy Patricia Bragg, "Vegetable Gourmet Recipes"

 Mock Mimosa

1 (32-oz) bottle white grape juice
4 cups orange juice
Squeeze of lime

Combine ingredients and serve chilled.

YIELDS: 2 QUARTS

Nutritional breakdown: 2 grams protein, 32 grams carbohydrate, 0 grams fat
Serving portion: 1 cup
Calories per serving: 134
Recipe courtesy Mandy Ganes

Hot Spiced Pineapple Tea

5 1/2 cups pineapple juice, unsweetened
1/4 cup honey
2 cinnamon sticks, broken
2 peppermint tea bags

1. In a saucepan, combine pineapple juice, honey, and cinnamon sticks. Bring to a boil; boil 1 minute. Remove from heat.
2. Add tea bags; steep 2 to 5 minutes.
3. Remove tea bags and cinnamon before serving. Garnish as desired.

YIELDS: 6 CUPS

Nutritional breakdown: 1 gram protein, 43 grams carbohydrate, 0 grams fat
Serving portion: 1 cup
Calories per serving: 176
Recipe courtesy Safeway, Inc., 1988

Snack hint: Slice bananas, sprinkle lightly with lemon juice, freeze the slices, and store for later use as a nutritious snack. Grapes also work well.

Good Snacks

11

◉ *Stuffed Celery*

2 (3-inch) celery ribs
1 tbsp natural peanut butter or almond
  butter
or
2 (3-inch) celery ribs
1 tbsp plain low-fat yogurt, sprinkled with
  vegetable salt
1 tbsp low-fat cottage cheese
or
2 (3-inch) celery ribs
2 tbsps caviar mixed with onion juice
or
2 (3-inch) celery ribs
2 fresh mushrooms, minced with 1 tsp
  horseradish
or
2 (3-inch) celery ribs
Imitation crabmeat

1. After cleaning thoroughly, cut celery into 3-inch lengths.
2. Press peanut butter or any filling into crook of celery. Serve.

YIELDS: 1 SERVING

Nutritional breakdown: 7 grams protein, 6 grams carbohydrate, 9 grams fat
Serving portion: 2 stuffed celery sticks
Calories per serving (based on peanut butter): 120

Tabasco Nuts

1 1/2 cups almonds or cashews
1 tbsp olive oil
1 to 2 tsps Tabasco sauce

1. Sauté almonds or cashews in olive oil until nuts are golden brown.
2. Remove from heat and sprinkle with Tabasco sauce.
3. Allow to cool.

YIELDS: 6 SERVINGS

Nutritional breakdown: 6 grams protein, 7 grams carbohydrate, 19 grams fat
Serving portion: 1/4 cup
Calories per serving: 211
Recipe courtesy Lucy Thomas, Louisiana Pacific Corp.

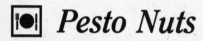

Pesto Nuts

1 cup shelled pecans
1 cup fresh basil leaves
3 garlic cloves
1/4 cup olive oil
3 tbsps grated Parmesan cheese
Freshly ground pepper

1. Cover pecans with boiling water and let stand for 30 minutes.
2. Drain thoroughly, then toast nuts for 30 minutes in a 350-degree oven on a cookie sheet lined with paper towels. Shake occasionally.
3. Mince basil and garlic together.
4. Sauté pecans in a preheated skillet coated with olive oil for about 5 minutes, or until nuts are shiny and coated with oil. Add basil mix and cook for 5 more minutes.
5. Sprinkle with cheese and pepper and sauté for another minute.
6. Allow to cool and store in an airtight container.

YIELDS: 6 SERVINGS

Nutritional breakdown: 3 grams protein, 4 grams carbohydrate, 13 grams fat
Serving portion: 1/6 recipe
Calories per serving: 139
Recipe courtesy Lucy Thomas, Louisiana Pacific Corp.

Jack's Frozen Fruit

When fresh fruits are in season, why not think about doing your own freezing so you can enjoy the fresh fruit when it's out of season?

3 cups fresh fruit in season (raspberries, strawberries, sliced peaches, blueberries, etc.)

1. Place fruits on a baking sheet, making certain they do not touch one another.
2. Place in freezer compartment.
3. When they are solidly frozen, place in freezer bags and stack in freezer. Be sure to mark freezer bags with the date you froze the fruit.
4. Take out and use when you get the urge to experience fruits out of season.

YIELDS: 3 CUPS

Nutritional breakdown: 0 grams protein, 7 grams carbohydrate, 0 grams fat
Serving portion: 1/2 cup
Calories per serving: 30

Fruitsicles

1 cup crushed pineapple, unsweetened
3 tbsps frozen orange juice concentrate
1 ripe banana
1 cup apple juice
1 tbsp dry milk powder (nonfat)

1. Process the ingredients in a blender.
2. Pour into paper cups and place in freezer.
3. When partially frozen, insert wooden sticks. You can also use the commercially available popsicle makers or use an ice cube tray.

Variation:

Add 1 tablespoon peanut butter to your mixture.

YIELDS: 3 CUPS

Nutritional breakdown: 2 grams protein, 32 grams carbohydrate, 0 grams fat
Serving portion: 1 fruitsicle
Calories per serving: 128

Broiled Potato Skins

1 medium russet potato
1 tsp safflower oil
1/2 tsp seasoning (pick one): garlic powder, vegetable seasoning, lemon pepper, fresh chives

1. Bake potato as usual.
2. When finished, cut potato in half lengthwise. Scoop out insides and save for another use.
3. Brush inside of potato skin with safflower oil and add your choice of seasonings.
4. Broil skin until crisp.

Hint:

Save potato pulp for potato burritos, potato pancakes, potato salad, or cube in green salad.

YIELDS: 1 SERVING

Nutritional breakdown: 2 grams protein, 17 grams carbohydrate, 2 grams fat
Serving portion: 1 skin
Calories per serving: 94

Rice Cake with Salsa

7 oz green chilies, thinly sliced
4 tomatoes, diced
1 large yellow onion, chopped
1 pkg rice cakes
1/2 cup plain nonfat yogurt

1. Combine all the ingredients except rice cakes and yogurt; season to taste.
2. Spread a thin layer of plain yogurt over rice cake and top with salsa mix.

YIELDS: 3 CUPS SALSA, 27 SERVINGS

Nutritional breakdown: 2 grams protein, 13 grams carbohydrate, 2 grams fat
Serving portion: 2 teaspoons yogurt, 2 tablespoons salsa, 1 rice cake
Calories per serving: 66
Recipe courtesy Ruth Allen

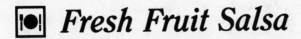 Fresh Veggies Dip

1/2 cup tomato purée
1/4 cup horseradish (or to taste)
2 tbsps minced onion
1/2 cup plain nonfat yogurt

1. Mix tomato purée, horseradish, and onion. Fold in yogurt.
2. Serve with assorted raw vegetables (such as cauliflower, broccoli, carrots, celery, jicama, etc.)

YIELDS: 1 1/4 CUPS

Nutritional breakdown: 0 grams protein, 1 gram carbohydrate, 0 grams fat
Serving portion: 1 tablespoon
Calories per serving: 6

Fresh Fruit Salsa

1 1/2 cups diced assorted fresh fruits (soft fruits, such as melons, berries, pineapple, etc.)
2 tbsps chopped fresh mint
1 tbsp lime juice
1/4 tsp grated lime rind

1. Mix all the ingredients, then let set for 2 to 3 hours.
2. Can be used for breakfast, lunch, dinner, any category. (Optional: Can be used over hot or cold cereal, over a half melon, over rice cakes, or as a general relish.)

YIELDS: 1 1/2 CUPS

Nutritional breakdown: 0 grams protein, 5 grams carbohydrate, 0 grams fat
Serving portion: 1/4 cup
Calories per serving: 20
Recipe courtesy Dr. Loriene Chase-King

🍽 Tasty Onion Rings

1 onion, sliced into 1/3-inch rings
2 tbsps vegetable oil
2 tbsps seasoned garlic powder
2 tsps vegetable salt
1 tsp lemon pepper

1. Line a baking sheet with aluminum foil. Dip onion rings in vegetable oil.
2. Combine seasonings in a small paper bag. Drop onion rings in and shake.
3. Place rings on baking sheet, but don't let them touch.
4. Bake at 450 degrees. Check after 15 minutes. They're ready when they're golden brown.

YIELDS: 3 SERVINGS

Nutritional breakdown: 0 gram protein, 5 grams carbohydrate, 9 grams fat
Serving portion: 1/3 recipe
Calories per serving: 101

🍽 Tofu Dip

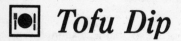

1/2 cup tofu
1/2 cup plain low-fat yogurt
1/4 tsp celery salt
1 tsp vegetable flakes
1/2 tsp parsley
1/2 tsp dill
1 tsp lemon juice

1. Mash tofu and add yogurt and seasonings.
2. Serve with zucchini spears and carrot sticks.

YIELDS: 1 CUP

Nutritional breakdown: 4 grams protein, 3 grams carbohydrate, 2 grams fat
Serving portion: 2 tablespoons
Calories per serving: 39

Bean Pesto Dip with Corn Chips

1 (16-oz) can kidney beans or black beans,
  drained
1/2 small jalapeño pepper (fresh or canned),
  sliced
1 or 2 garlic cloves (to taste)
1 dozen corn tortillas
Vegetable salt or seasoned salt

1. Process beans, jalapeño, and garlic in a blender or food processor until smooth.
2. Cut each tortilla into 8 triangles.
3. Place on a vegetable-sprayed baking sheet and bake about 5 minutes, or until crispy. If desired, turn chips over and crisp other side.
4. Sprinkle with vegetable salt or seasoned salt.
5. Cool and store in an airtight container. Serve with bean pesto dip.

Variation:

After blending, add 1 teaspoon chili powder and/or 1 teaspoon cumin to tone down jalapeño.

Hint:

Jalapeño peppers are known for their hotness, so add slices one at a time until you reach a taste suitable for you.

YIELDS: 1 1/2 CUPS PESTO AND 96 CHIPS

Nutritional breakdown: 4 grams protein, 19 grams carbohydrate, 1 gram fat
Serving portion: 2 tablespoons pesto and 8 chips
Calories per serving: 103

Revive the flavor of dried herbs by soaking in a bit of lemon juice.

Mary's Mother's Armenian Dolma (Stuffed Grape Leaves)

5 cups diced onions
3/4 cup olive oil (reserve 1/4 cup for simmering)
1 cup rice (uncooked)
1 cup chopped parsley
1 tsp salt
1 (8-oz) can tomato sauce
1 jar grape leaves
1 1/2 cups water
2 lemons

1. In a large frying pan, sauté onions in 1/2 cup oil.
2. Add uncooked rice, parsley, salt, and tomato sauce. Cook on a low burner until almost tender. Stir occasionally to prevent sticking.
3. Gently remove grape leaves from jar and drain in a colander. Use any torn pieces to line the top and bottom of a large saucepan. Put 1 tablespoon of rice mixture on each grape leaf. Roll and fold. Place the dolma snugly on the bottom of lined saucepan. Continue to stack until pan is about three quarters full. Lay remaining leaves and leaf pieces on top to cover. Sprinkle with salt. Add reserved 1/4 cup olive oil and 1 1/2 cups water.
4. Place a saucer or small plate (inverted) on top to hold dolmas in place. Cover and simmer until water is all cooked away, 30 to 45 minutes.
5. Turn off heat, remove inverted plate, sprinkle with juice of 1 lemon, and re-cover with plate. Let stand to cool.
6. To serve, place slices of lemon on top of dolmas and arrange on a platter.

Hints:

1. May also be baked in the oven. Using a deep covered casserole, bake at 350 degrees 45 to 60 minutes.
2. Leftovers keep well in the refrigerator for up to 2 weeks.

YIELDS: 24 DOLMAS

Nutritional breakdown: 4 grams protein, 30 grams carbohydrate, 21 grams fat
Serving portion: 3 dolmas
Calories per serving: 317
Recipe courtesy Mary Robertson

Index

A

B

T

Tabasco Nuts, 158
Tamale Pie, Raechel's, 98
Tangy Pocket Burgers, 90
Tannins, 34
Tart, Jewel Fruit, 143
Tasty Onion Rings, 162
Tea, 25, 34, 41, 52
　Alfalfa, 150
　Bread, Carolyn's English, 141
　Fruit, 153
　Hot Spiced Pineapple, 156
　Lemon and Barley, 150
Teeth, 52, 53
Thiamin, 48
Thirst, 37
Throat cancer, 34
Thyme Carrots, 123
Toast, Banana, 79
Tobacco, 32
To do list, 66
Tofu
　Dip, 162
　Patty, 92
　Reliable Rice Pudding, 132
　Rounds in Sauce, 116
Tomatoes
　Ratatouille, 119
　Roast Stuffed Leg of Lamb with
　　Broiled, 108
　Sauce
　　for Cabbage, 104
　　Fresh, 102
　　Off-the-Shelf Pasta, 113
　　Rice Cake with Salsa, 160
　　Spaghetti Sauce for an Army, 103
Tongue (as food), 20
Toxic
　effects of vitamins, 46–47
　metabolites, 27
Triglyceride levels, 24
Tropical Sherbert, 134
Trout, 19
Tuna, 20
　Broiled or Barbecued, 111
　Jon's Tempting Salad, 83
　Off-the-Shelf Pasta, 113
　Sushi, 92

Turkey, 18, 20
　Cranberry Cutlets, 102
　Elaine's Stuffed Cabbage, 104
　Loaf, Eric's Tantalizing, 101
　skin, 19
　Soup, 106
　Spaghetti Sauce for an Army,
　　103
　Surprise Meatballs, 105
　Swinger, 106
　Wheat Chili, 105
Turnips, 32
12-Minute Oatmeal Cookies, 138

U

Upside-Down Gingerbread, 148
Urinary tract cancer, 33
Urine, 26, 28, 37

V

Vascular disease, 38
Veal, 18
　cuts to avoid, 19
　Stew, 107
Vegetables, 32, 34, 35, 36
　Be-Fit Beverage, 154
　cooking, 12, 13
　Fresh Veggies and Dip, 161
　Jack's Chop-Chop with Spaghetti and
　　Chicken, 97
　Lasagne, 115
　Meatless Chili, 116
　Pasta Vegetarian, 82
　Ratatouille, 119
　Soup
　　Jack's Blender, 85
　　Turkey, 106
　Steak and Veggies, 107
　Tofu Rounds in Sauce, 116
　See also specific vegetables
Vinegar, Raspberry, 81
Vitamin A, 47, 53
Vitamin and mineral supplements,
　　16–17, 44–48, 53, 54
　guidelines for choosing, 47–48